Comments on

Diabetes Through the Looking Glass

from readers

I think the book is an inspiration to worried parents like myself and provides a great deal of comfort on how to address the many challenges facing a parent when raising a child with Type 1. It is much appreciated.

Howard Lack, whose son aged 11 was diagnosed at 9 years

I wish this book had been available when my son was diagnosed. Dr Besser presents a clear, accessible account of Type 1 diabetes from the child's point of view, which is why this is such an important book and such a marvellous resource for parents. What's more, she includes an array of children's views — after all no two cases are the same — and draws together the gems of wisdom in a sensible, reassuring fashion. This is a must for parents and children alike.

Dai Williams, Diabetes UK National Director, Wales, and whose son aged 19 was diagnosed at 13 years

I love this book! I cried and laughed out loud. If others, like me, regard the book *Type 1 Diabetes in children, adolescents and young adults* by Ragnar Hanas as their diabetes Bible, then this book should become their Book of Common Prayer. It is full of the everyday cares and concerns of all those in a family who are affected by diabetes, and offers practical suggestions on ways you can tackle even the most intimate of issues.

Jacqui Double, whose children aged 8 and 9 were diagnosed at 18 months

We could really have done with a book like this when our son was first diagnosed.

Kate Evans, whose son aged 9 was diagnosed at 3 years

Firstly let me say how user-friendly the book is; this is real life diabetes written by someone with personal knowledge and insight, and who understands the diabetes journey. There is no hiding the fact that diabetes is a maze where people may find themselves taking the wrong path, but with the right support they can eventually find their way. Rachel Besser has written the truth and the pictures and words from the children and adults are real, and add to the richness of the book.

Jo Butler, diabetes consultant nurse, and whose daughter aged 16 was diagnosed at 11 years

I can't wait to let my family read it. A book like this is needed in my life.

Michael Brown, aged 18, diagnosed at 12 years

In the consulting room the pressing need to cover medical information means that the emotional impact is often passed over. By presenting the child's viewpoint so clearly, Rachel Besser answers many of the questions that parents will ask and provides a wealth of useful information and helpful advice on everyday management.

Kate Fazakerley, whose daughter aged 11 was diagnosed at 2 years

This book is inspirational. It shows to everybody associated with diabetes that there is light at the end of the tunnel.

Nigel Jenner, aged 37, diagnosed at 3 years

Reviews of
Diabetes Through the Looking Glass

We think this is a really great, informative book. It echoes so many of the thoughts from parents and children I have heard while working at JDRF. It is very hard for those of us without Type 1 diabetes to have any concept of what children, and adults with Type 1, and their families deal with every day, but this goes a long way to improving that understanding.

Sarah Johnson, Director of Policy and Communications, Juvenile Diabetes Research Foundation

This is a book of pearls. It is all relevant, real and wise. A lot of thinking has gone into it.

Dr Charles Fox, Consultant Physician with Special Interest in Diabetes

I find it quite fascinating reading with a great insight into the mysteries of being a child, a teenager and a young adult with diabetes.

Dr Ragnar Hanas, Consultant Paediatrician

For Mum, Dad and J
– for everything

Diabetes Through the Looking Glass

Seeing diabetes from your child's perspective

Dr Rachel Besser

BSc MBBS (Hons) MRCPCH

CLASS PUBLISHING · LONDON

Text © Rachel Besser, 2009
Typography © Class Publishing Ltd, 2009

Printing history
First published 2009

The author and publishers welcome feedback from the users of this
book. Please contact the publishers.

Class Publishing Ltd, Barb House, Barb Mews, London W6 7PA, UK
Telephone: 020 7371 2119
Fax: 020 7371 2878 [International +4420]
email: post@class.co.uk
Website: www.class.co.uk

A CIP catalogue for this book is available from the British Library

ISBN 978 1 85959 209 0
10 9 8 7 6 5 4 3 2 1

616.462
BES

Edited by Caroline Sheldrick

Illustrations by David Woodroffe

Cover illustration based on an original drawing by Louis Blatherwick,
aged 11

Designed and typeset by Ray Rich

Printed and bound in Finland by WS Bookwell, Juva

Contents

Foreword

This is a very special book in the sense that you will find both detailed information on how to take care of your child's diabetes, and people sharing how it is to live with diabetes. Add to this the view of Dr Rachel Besser, a paediatric specialist who herself has had Type 1 diabetes since childhood. I find it fascinating reading, giving great insight into the mysteries of being a child, a teenager and a young adult with diabetes. Rachel takes you through the different phases of diagnosis, dealing with hypoglycemia, the anatomy of your pancreas, different types of insulin and many more topics. She explains difficult things like 'hypoglycemia unawareness' (feeling your hypoglycaemia symptoms at a lower blood glucose level than usual) in simple words that you will recognise and understand. She gives balanced advice to parents of children with diabetes in different situations from having sweets to going on school trips.

Children, adolescents and parents give their view on a lot of topics and problems, and it is encouraging to find how they deal with their diabetes in the most varying ways, always seeming to find their way out safely. You will even find some good things about having diabetes, like 'When my friends were smoking I used my diabetes as an excuse not to start'. You will learn a lot of tips and tricks about travelling with diabetes from young people who have done it, and share their ways of success in handling trips lasting a day or a year. The bothersome times of high blood sugars and ketone levels are dealt with in detail, and the troublesome thoughts on long-term complications are met with a Question and Answers session. There are many quotes from people from 8 to 37 years of age. As you can imagine, their views differ a lot, but there is a true story in every one, and it should be comforting for someone new to diabetes to read these honest comments.

Food and diabetes are closely linked, and for some teenagers and young adults, eating disorders have been become a demanding part of their everyday life. Rachel describes this in honest and straightforward wording, and the people who are interviewed share their insight and information with you in a way that is really touching.

Bringing up a child with diabetes is not easy. On the other hand, bringing up a child without diabetes is difficult at times too. Here you will find answers to many of the questions that relate to diabetes, but also get simple and seemingly obvious advice like 'Would you tell her off if she didn't have diabetes?'

Is your child in school? Does he or she get the extra attention needed to perform well? Rachel covers the legal aspects and gives good advice on how to meet and inform the school staff.

How are siblings affected by the necessary extra attention that the child with diabetes gets? Learn from children and parents sharing their own experiences.

What happens during the years of teenage liberation? How do you tell a girl- or a boyfriend about your diabetes? The young people in this book generously share their thoughts on all kinds of topics that are familiar in everyday life.

In the latter part of the book Rachel moves from the teenage years to life beyond home. This was very interesting reading for me and she has really made a great catch of what the experts with diabetes themselves feel and think. This is very informative for someone having diabetes, but also imparts important knowledge and insight for their friends, spouses and workmates. It is also valuable to healthcare workers. Whether you are a doctor, diabetes nurse, dietitian, psychologist, teacher who comes into contact with people who have diabetes, here is your chance of a real understanding of how it really is to live with diabetes. I truly recommend this book to everyone who wants to increase their understanding of diabetes.

Ragnar Hanas, MD, PhD

Ragnar Hanas is a Consultant Paediatrician at the Department of Paediatrics, Uddevalla Hospital, Uddevalla, Sweden. He is co-editor of the 2009 ISPAD Clinical Practice Consensus Guidelines, and is the current Secretary General of ISPAD (International Society for Paediatric and Adolescent Diabetes).

Acknowledgements

My thanks go to everyone who has helped me give children and adults with diabetes a voice. This book could never have been written without the contribution of many children, young people and adults with diabetes, their parents, brothers and sisters. I would like to thank them all for trusting me with their personal stories, drawings and poems.

I owe a great debt of thanks to Peter Sönksen for the book's title, the encouragement to go forward and for reading the first draft of each chapter.

Special mention go to the following: Bruce Fogle for helping me to identify the subject of the book and his encouragement; Susan Grossman and Wendy Perriam, who always told me I could do it; Mary MacKinnon for her advice, support and enthusiasm; Jeannette Josse for clarification of the psychological issues; Dorothy Garvie, who has been a brilliant mentor since I was a medical student and has encouraged me with each chapter; Martin Savage for giving me such a good start and Diabetes UK and the JDRF for their endorsements.

I would also like to thank all those who read and gave me honest feedback on all of the early raw chapters, in particular Peter Sönksen, Charles Fox, Sharon March, Tracy Lee, Neil and Kate Evans, Katie Hopgood, Nigel Jenner and my Mum and Dad as well as the reviewers who read and improved upon the final proofs: Ragnar Hanas, Charles Fox, Jacqui Double, Kate Fazakerley, Jo Butler, Howard Lack and Dai Williams. If I have inadvertently omitted anyone, it is no reflection on my gratitude, merely the result of pressure from working full-time and writing a book at the same time.

The team at Class showed much patience and understanding during the editing of the book, for which I am extremely grateful. To my family and to all my friends who have put up with me and egged me on: thank you!

I would like to acknowledge the International Society for Paediatric and Adolescent Diabetes (ISPAD), whose guidelines were extremely useful in clarifying and supporting the medical facts in the book.

Last, but most importantly for me, Edwin Gale deserves a hug of thanks, for always believing in me.

Introduction

It was when I was diagnosed with Type 1 diabetes, at 9 years of age, that I decided to become a paediatrician. Twenty-three years later, despite spending six years at medical school and working since as a doctor, it is mostly through living with diabetes that I have come to understand the condition. Even now, however, my diabetes surprises me and catches me out.

Many books describe the technicalities of managing diabetes in childhood, but none of them fully embrace the emotional aspects that come hand-in-hand with living with diabetes.

The idea for this book came from participating in many diabetes children's camps and family support weekends over the years. One session always involves a panel of adults who had Type 1 diabetes in childhood answering questions from parents. The questions are always a variation on similar themes: What does it feel like to have a hypo? Did you blame your parents for your diabetes? Has your diabetes ever stopped you doing anything? Have you ever been discriminated against? When is the right time to talk about complications?

Ultimately, parents yearn to understand how it feels for their child to live with diabetes and worry whether they will grow up to lead a normal life. They struggle to achieve a balance between good diabetes control and allowing their child to grow up normally. Parents may not realise that there are certain questions which, if asked, could explain their child's feelings and behaviour.

Sometimes the path to asking a child those questions is littered with obstacles. The question might be too sensitive or too difficult emotionally for the parent or child to cope with, or perhaps the child is too young to give a verbal response. Parents rarely get the opportunity to ask such questions, since most of their interaction with diabetes comes with things like persuading their child to eat just one more spoonful of mashed potato to avoid a night hypo, or to have their injection, not just today, but for ever; or trying to figure out why their child's blood sugar is 16.5 mmol/l before supper – did they have enough insulin, or did they eat some sweets on the way home from school?

I only realised when working with families just how much diabetes affects the whole family and the devastation that a diagnosis can bring. It can tip you all upside down. Sometimes parents blame themselves. Parents as well as children worry about the future. Often the family is caught up in a constant battle over blood testing, injection time and food. Alternatively the child may appear accepting and placid and the parent often wonders what their child is feeling inside.

Understanding what it feels like to have diabetes, or rather, not understanding what it feels like, can lead to frustration and isolation. Many children and families do not know anyone else with diabetes and can feel utterly alone. There is a wealth of books which explain about diabetes and how to manage it. However, there are none explaining to parents what it really feels like to grow up with diabetes. To redress the balance, I hope in this book to share some of my own and others' experiences from diagnosis in childhood to the emergence into adult life, which will be a unique insight and true Diabetes Through the Looking Glass.

I hope that understanding what it feels like to live with diabetes from your child's perspective will help you to understand why your child behaves in a certain way. I hope, too, that this book gives you, your child, their brothers and sisters, wider family and friends the confidence to talk to each other, and that it will generate discussion between you, and you will find your own answers.

Before you start reading, I must stress that this book is based on how diabetes felt to me whilst growing up, and my contact with others with diabetes including those whom I have formally and informally interviewed. I have worried at length that I may not have included a representative sample. However, by definition that would be impossible since diabetes is unique to each individual.

I hope any difficulties you encounter or worries you may have will be discussed in the following pages.

If you really want to know what it feels like for your own child to be living with Type 1 diabetes, you will have to ask them.

1

Diagnosis, getting real and getting on

What is diabetes?

Diabetes develops when there is not enough insulin around to keep the body's blood glucose levels within normal limits, which is around 5 mmol/l. Glucose is a type of sugar that we get from certain foods. Glucose is packaged as glycogen which is stored in the liver and used when needed for energy. Apart from particular foods, blood glucose can also be raised by a variety of hormones – these are the body's chemical messengers which are released into the bloodstream – one of which is called glucagon. There are several hormones that may raise blood glucose, but only one, insulin, which can lower blood glucose. So if there is no insulin around, blood glucose levels remain high even if no glucose-containing food is eaten.

Blood glucose regulation

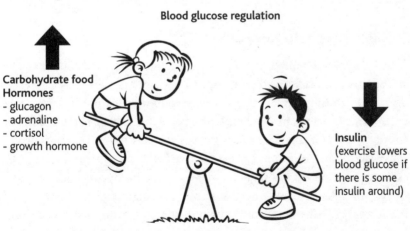

Carbohydrate food
Hormones
- glucagon
- adrenaline
- cortisol
- growth hormone

Insulin
(exercise lowers blood glucose if there is some insulin around)

Blood glucose will remain high if no insulin is around, even if no carbohydrates or glucose-containing food are eaten

The balancing system that normally regulates insulin production

1

One of the important jobs of insulin is to regulate how much glucose is produced by the liver, both from breakdown of glycogen stores as well as forming new glucose. The balance between glucagon which raises blood glucose, and insulin which lowers it, controls how much glucose is produced by the liver to such a fine degree as to keep the blood glucose constant at around 5mmol/l, slightly more after eating. This sounds a bit like a see-saw, which it is, but a very sophisticated one.

Without insulin, muscle and fat are also broken down. The breakdown products are used to make the new glucose in the liver and produce ketones, which are chemicals that make the blood more acidic than normal. They also cause tummy pain, feeling sick, vomiting, lack of appetite and even confusion. Ketones are produced in the liver when there is not enough sugar available. At low levels in the blood they are a good source of spare energy that can be used, for example, by the brain or the heart.

In 'Type 1' (previously known as 'insulin-dependent') diabetes, which mostly occurs in children and young adults, there is an almost complete lack of insulin. In 'Type 2' (previously know as 'non-insulin dependent') diabetes, which usually occurs in older people, less commonly in children, insulin is present but the body is resistant to it regulating the body's blood glucose. There are other forms of diabetes which can affect children but these are even rarer (see www.diabetes genes.org for more information).

What causes diabetes?

Type 1 diabetes is thought to result from a combination of someone's genes and an unknown factor in the environment, which may be a virus. Our genes determine all the characteristics which we inherit from our parents. An environmental factor, in someone with a particular genetic make-up, sets up a series of body reactions over several weeks, months or even years, which cause the body's immune system to attack the insulin-producing cells, causing them to stop working and therefore stop producing insulin. This is why people refer to diabetes as an autoimmune condition, *auto* meaning self. It also explains why the identical twin of someone with diabetes, with the same genetic make-up, has only a 36% chance of developing diabetes too.

The body's insulin-producing cells are called beta cells and are found in part of the pancreas called the islets of Langerhans. The pancreas is an organ which lies behind the stomach. There may be some insulin being produced at diagnosis but not enough to do its job of regulating blood glucose properly. After starting to take insulin, the beta cells may 'rest' for a while and then become able to start producing more insulin. Insulin requirements are likely to fall at this time and blood glucose levels become relatively easy to control, although you may only realise this with hindsight. This is why it is called the 'honeymoon phase'. However, this usually only lasts for a few months, rarely more than 2 years, after which the beta cells stop making insulin altogether.

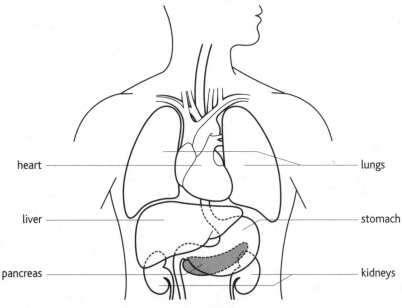

heart   lungs

liver   stomach

pancreas   kidneys

The position of the pancreas

How common is diabetes?

Type 1 diabetes affects approximately 1 in every 1000 of all children in developed countries, although this varies greatly between countries. There has been an increase in Type 1 diabetes in many countries, especially in children under the age of 5 years. Over 97% of children in the UK with diabetes have Type 1.

What tests show a child has diabetes?

A blood test will show how high the blood glucose level is. A urine test may show glucose in the urine if the blood glucose level is high enough to cause it to spill over into the urine. When glucose levels in the blood are high and lots of glucose is in the urine, the body also loses water and becomes dry (dehydrated). This would make someone feel thirsty as well as pass urine more than usual. Ketones, which are what make children with diabetes unwell, are most commonly measured in the urine but can also be measured in blood.

Just before I was diagnosed we had to draw the perfect meal in school. Mine was a monumentous orange juice.

(Jason, 27, diagnosed aged 7)

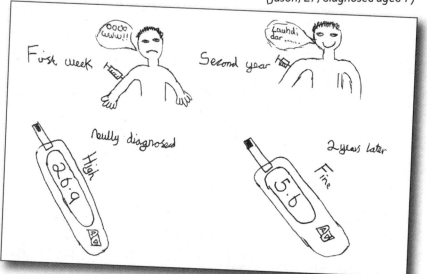

A boy of 11 shows how much has changed in the year
since his diagnosis

Case 1

A daughter and mother remember when diabetes arrived in their lives

Introducing Lizzie, 27, diagnosed aged 8

I remember being thirsty all the time, no matter how much I drank and I was wetting the bed at night. I was so embarrassed and hid what was happening. I would wake up in the night with a wet bed and creep out to the bathroom to get a towel to lie on for the rest of the night.

Case 1 *continued*

One day after school, Mum took me in the car to the hospital. I remember my last memories of not having diabetes. I was talking to Mum in our beige Mini in the front seat. I remember feeling hungry and craving a Mars bar.

In the hospital I had to wee into a pot and have a blood test. I sat outside while the doctor talked to Mum and Dad, feeling tired and wanting to go home. I went inside the doctor's room and sat on Dad's knee. I don't really remember what Dad said except when he told me I couldn't eat sweets any more. That's when I cried. It made him cry too so I stopped myself crying as I didn't want to upset him. I'd never seen my Dad cry before.

I stayed in hospital for a week after that. I enjoyed getting loads of presents. My brother gave me his whole *Beano* collection, although I had to give it back when I came out of hospital.

Lizzie's mum remembers

I remember when Lizzie was diagnosed as if it were yesterday. I asked myself, 'What have I done wrong?' As a parent, you want your children to be perfect and have a perfect life. I felt as if I'd let her down and had given her an extra burden to carry throughout her life. From the beginning we knew we had to help her do as much as she could for herself. Now I know that diabetes is just something that happened and that it was not my fault and I see how wonderfully she has coped. I had to hang in there and hang onto myself, as I wouldn't have been able to help her if I'd shown her how I felt. You get used to your fears and worries and they get easier. You learn that diabetes is a manageable condition and nothing need stand in the way.

Discussion

Lizzie describes the classic symptoms leading up to a diagnosis, that of thirst and frequent passing of urine. She knew something was wrong but didn't know what, hiding the fact that she was wetting the bed at night. When the news was broken to Lizzie about her diagnosis, the shock was the 'no sweets'. That is a common memory of diagnosis. Many people still have the false belief that if you have diabetes you are not able to eat sweets at all, but sweets are not 'poisonous' to people with diabetes. Apart from that, Lizzie remembers the presents, although she wasn't sure why she'd got them.

Once Lizzie saw her dad crying she hid her own tears, so upset at having been the cause of her father being sad. Lizzie's mum also hid her real feelings from Lizzie, sparing her further stress and worry but also carrying an extra burden herself.

If this is what you do, it will be important that you have support and be able to let your feelings out in some way, otherwise they may build up inside. Your child will be able to pick up on your feelings, however hard you try to hide them.

Talking to Lizzie's parents about the time when she was diagnosed, they recollected a slightly different sequence of events to Lizzie. Having taken Lizzie home after misunderstanding instructions by the doctor in the hospital, they had to bring her back where she was admitted onto the Children's Ward. Lizzie does not remember how ill she must have felt, described by her parents to me as having 'hollowed out eyes' and having 'lost a lot of weight'. Clearly it was a traumatic experience for Lizzie's parents having to watch her go on an intravenous drip and then face up to her diagnosis. What you experience as parents is often far worse than it is for your child. Most parents will remember where you were, the date, time and even what clothes you were wearing at the time of diagnosis. This may explain why you react the way you do, worrying a lot of the time. Some of you may even feel you are turning into 'the nag', worrying about your child being unwell.

Lizzie's mother describes her guilt and disappointment at the loss of her 'perfect' child. Some of what you may feel, interwoven with the natural guilt and blame, may relate to your worries about what the future may hold. Often these worries are outdated, as things have moved on a lot both in terms of insulin management and the prevention and treatment of complications. However, they may add to your fear and anger. With time, experience and wisdom, Lizzie's mum realised she was not to blame, whilst from the wings she could watch her fly.

When your child is diagnosed with diabetes, so are you. At the beginning, everything may seem a big issue and your life may seem to revolve around diabetes. You may even feel resentful of all the time you use just on diabetes, away from the rest of your family. It needn't always be like this.

Case 2

A young person remembers

Introducing Daniel, 17, diagnosed aged 12

I was first diagnosed with a urine infection. Ten seconds after I had a drink I had to rush to the toilet. It was going on for weeks. When they did my blood sugar it was in the 30s. Then everything's a blur until I'm sitting on the hospital ward bed. The nurse is with me. She's explaining how diabetes is going to affect my life – it's carbohydrate control and eat less sugar. It seemed to me I could never eat a sweet again. It was a bit of a shock, even though I didn't eat a lot of sweets, to never eat sweets again.

I was being taught how to use a Novopen [pen injection device] and how to do a blood test. I was holding my Mum's hand and looking away and she injected me in my leg.

Discussion

Daniel was probably wrongly diagnosed as having a urine infection as he needed to pass urine frequently. Some of you may have similarly experienced a delayed diagnosis, especially if your child is young.

Daniel remembers two main things about his diagnosis: being told he couldn't eat sweets and his first injection. His mum was with him and they shared the experience together. It is important to allow family members to help, both in supporting you and your child as well as sharing your and your child's first experiences. If you have a partner it will be important for both parents to be there as much as possible to share experiences from the beginning. If you are a single parent, allowing family members and friends to share with you will ease your anxiety and mean that later down the line you will need to explain things less, and you and your child will feel more supported.

This will also help to avoid feeling as if one of you has taken on all of the diabetes care, which can feel like a frightening responsibility at the beginning. After a while diabetes will hopefully become part of your daily routine.

Case 3

A young person remembers

Introducing Juliet, 22, diagnosed aged 17

I was diagnosed with my diabetes when I was 17, just as I was going into upper sixth, the time when we had to decide what Unis we wanted to go to. At first I remember crying to my Mum because I was scared about coping with my diabetes on my own. In the hospital I was given a book to read. It kept saying that you couldn't do this and you couldn't do that. I was really scared. My doctor said her daughter went to college and stayed out late – 'but you won't be doing that'; that she drank alcohol in the college bar 'but you won't be doing that'. I was about to go off to college and I thought that I wouldn't be able to do any of those things, that my life was ruined. Now I see her in clinic. She sits behind her desk. I think, 'You have no idea'.

My parents are very supportive with my diabetes. When I first got out of hospital and had to deal with my diabetes with no nurses and doctors around, my Mum was key and there for me every step of the way.

Discussion

Often what a child remembers about their diagnosis may be different from the sequence of events that happened and what was actually said, or they may remember something that was said unintentionally. The light-hearted throwaway comment by a healthcare professional or relative may be the only thing that a child, or a parent, remembers. They can carry this with them forever. I wonder in Juliet's case whether what the doctor said, or intended to say, and the way Juliet perceived it was the same. I would hope not. Perhaps the doctor was trying to make light of the situation. However, it was clearly misjudged as Juliet was left feeling frightened and her experience of healthcare professionals in managing her diabetes had already caused mistrust. This would have the potential to damage their relationship in the future, and all in the first few days of diagnosis.

As in the previous cases, Juliet's mum was there from the beginning. However, Juliet describes 'her' diabetes, as many people with diabetes do. Even though you provide a lot of care, support, reminders and meals, it is still your child's diabetes. The sooner they can take ownership of it, when it is at the right time for them, the better. You may find it difficult to hand over control. It may make you feel less certain of the future. However, for your child, it means they can have a future that is independent and confident, like Juliet. It is a difficult balance to strike between being over-involved as a parent on the one hand and being neglectful on the other.

I have fond memories of the old Children's Hospital Ward. There was a huge playroom which I loved escaping into every day and there was a tiny room where we had classes, reading Peter and Jane books and making my Mum's Mother's Day card, which she kept for many years.

(Rebecca, 35, diagnosed aged 6)

Case 4

Getting real and getting on

Introducing Nigel, 37, diagnosed aged 3

I remember when I was diagnosed, even though I was only three. I was in hospital. Everyone was crying. I thought it was great – I was bought a big red toy tractor, it was fantastic. And it was the week before Christmas, so that was on top of more presents.

I've never used my diabetes as an excuse. Other people have tried to. Mum used to say, 'We have to go to the front of the queue.' I'd wince and absolutely hated it.

When I was playing rugby if the other team saw me doing a blood

continued on next page

Case 4 *continued*

test and knew I was diabetic, they thought they'd beaten me before I'd started. So when I nailed them and had diabetes the victory was even greater. At the back of my mind I knew having diabetes was a bit of a disadvantage, but I turned it into a positive.

It motivated me and gave me focus to ensure that my blood tests were good otherwise I'd get pulped on the pitch. Others probably didn't think those things at all but it was what I focused on. I was competing against them [the other team] but also against my diabetes.

I've never seriously thought I'm different to anyone else. I forget I've got diabetes. It's like I have a split personality; there's me and a person hovering in the background who's evil and has diabetes. I'm always trying to fend him off and show him it's [diabetes] not going to stop me doing anything. If you accept it, you become 'the diabetic' and I never wanted to be that. It doesn't bother me if I am called a diabetic, but I don't want to be 'the diabetic' of other people's perceptions. People always have preconceived ideas. Every person is an ambassador for the rest of us. I have anger at other people with diabetes who let the rest of us down. There's nothing complicated about beating the world with diabetes. You can't go on feeling sorry for yourself. Everyone goes through some sort of rebellion. Then you have to move on from it or diabetes rules your life.

Discussion

Nigel was able to use his competitive drive as a focus with his diabetes. As a result he also had good control, as he didn't want erratic blood glucose levels to get in his way. He never wanted to be or to feel different because of his diabetes. He did of course, but only because he has achieved so much (read about Nigel in Who's who, p.274). Having proven to himself and his fellow rugby team and opponents that diabetes didn't affect him in spite of assumed misconceptions, he is critical of others who use diabetes as an excuse. Nigel had a motivation to achieve good blood glucose control, otherwise he would be 'pulped' on the rugby field. He was in a regular routine at school with exercise and eating to maintain his fitness and this provided a template to get things spot on. Others may not have this motivation. Although the motivation required sounds harder, actually it can make life easier because there are other things to focus on rather than the diabetes, getting out there and living a life as well as having a routine that can be perfected.

Children innately push boundaries and this may be a reason for their excuses, to see what they can get away with. There are a whole variety of excuses children, young people and adults use when it comes to their diabetes. You can read about these in Chapter 11: The best and worst of times. Sometimes others offer up excuses to the person with diabetes and this introduces the idea to them that they are different. Children may pick up on your worries and because they unconsciously don't want to upset you, they may offer up an excuse not to do something. Nigel's method instead was, in his words, 'to use it as a motivation to get out there and kick some butt'.

Case 5

A parent remembers and finds hope

When Maeve was diagnosed, I felt totally devastated and cheated. My perfect little 7-year-old had just been afflicted with this awful disability, which I just wanted to give back straight away. Having worked in intensive care for more than 20 years as a nurse, diabetes to me meant terrible medical problems. We were discharged from the hospital on New Year's Day with a bag containing some leaflets, a blood testing kit and insulin, all geared up for a lifetime of injections and blood tests and left to it. We were petrified and devastated. How would we get through the weekend? We lay down on the sofa together and I cried my heart out and wished out loud that if only it could be me and not my beautiful little 7-year-old.

After a difficult few weeks of chasing her around the house for blood tests and injections things calmed down and life with diabetes became a reality. I was so elated one day at work when I got my handover and was told, 'In bed 6 is Mr Smith, 93-year-old

continued on next page

Case 5 *continued*

with suspected heart attack. History of Type 1 diabetes since childhood, otherwise no relevant history. Had been doing own injections until two weeks ago when district nurses came in to help.'

Mr Smith died soon after in a dignified manner but I will never forget him. He gave me hope, and I realised that if Maeve looked after herself she could be a Mrs Smith in 86 years' time.

We are so lucky to have a great local team of diabetic nurses and doctors. Maeve (now 9 years old) can live a fulfilled life. She is a happy and well-adjusted child coping with diabetes.

Discussion

Maeve's mum may describe some of what you felt when your child was diagnosed. It didn't help that she had some inside knowledge; she still went into shock and started grieving for herself and her child. She felt helpless and didn't know what to do to make things right again. In time, she and Maeve are learning to cope and make diabetes part of all their family's lives.

Here are recollections of other parents' experiences around the time of diagnosis.

❝ The paediatric consultant tried to explain to us about diabetes and drew graphs with peaks and lines. In spite of being well-educated and I suppose of average intelligence, I had no idea what he was talking about. I think I was numb in every sense. It wasn't until we got home and I read a book for children which spelt it out in very basic language, that I even started to grasp what it was all about. ❞

❝ In the early stages we worried a lot. I remember making my daughter cry as I sat with a snack by her bedside making her eat. I remember shouting at my husband when he forgot a snack. ❞

' The consultant took me to a room to tell me that my daughter (aged 4) had diabetes. He was lovely and sat massaging her feet whilst he explained everything to me. It still seemed like something I could easily cope with at this stage. She wasn't impressed with the injections but didn't fuss too much. The next morning I had a chat with the diabetic nurse; so much information and you couldn't do it in stages, you needed most of it now so we could go home. On the one hand I needed to know everything but on the other my brain was full, diabetes doesn't go away and I would have to do this for a very long time. It has taken me about 6 months to get my head into a 'managing' rather than a controlling way of thinking and to realise that actually we are doing OK. '

' I walked into the doctor's surgery and within 5 minutes was told that my little boy had a life-long medical condition that couldn't be 'fixed'. We coped by going into automatic pilot because we had to learn how to test his blood and do his injections – he was only two-and-a-half and needed us to look after him. I was numb. Everything in our lives seemed the same and yet completely different. I cried a lot. I was so angry that my beautiful little boy had been given this to deal with for the rest of his life – it just didn't feel fair. Usually when you leave hospital you go home well, but we had to take this illness with us. '

' When I think back to the early days of diagnosis it was a very bleak time. Only now do I know that things do work and how things work for us. In the early days it wasn't like that and it doesn't need to be. '

' I remember the call that my daughter may have diabetes as though it was yesterday. The following day when the diagnosis was confirmed I tried not to accept it thinking that there must be some mistake, diabetes doesn't run in our family so I didn't want to accept the diagnosis as being correct. I also hoped that it could be controlled through diet. There was no time for denial, however, and we were pushed straight into living with diabetes. We coped because we had to cope, there was no easing our way gently into things – once diagnosis is complete that's that! I felt awful, not for me but for my daughter who would now have to live with this for the rest of her life. Was this because of something I had done? I don't think I'm a bad person but was she paying for my shortcomings, should I have striven to be a better person, is this payback for something I have done wrong? I wanted so very much to share my wife and daughter's tears but felt that as the father I should show strength and assurance so I cried when I was alone. It still chokes me up when I think of my lovely daughter and the way she copes with the worry and constant thinking about diabetes management. My view of diabetes has changed considerably since then. I understand it a lot better now and it is no longer the monster I feared it to be. ⟩

Poem 1
Rufus the bear

Hey, hey, hey it's Rufus the bear,
Back with something new to share,
He says that he now has diabetes,
All that he wanted was to eat his sweeties.

Everyone says they'll find a cure,
Something original and something pure,
Rufus has 2 injections a day,
And in bed is where he had to stay.

Eating food with lots to do,
But now he keeps needing the loo,
Rufus is better now and wishes to tell,
The children with diabetes that he wishes them well.

A poem by a 13-year-old girl, about Rufus the Bear with Type 1 Diabetes. Rufus is part of the KIDSAC programme available to every child with Type 1 diabetes from Juvenile Diabetes Research Foundation.

Q **Is there any right way of telling my child she has diabetes?**

A No matter what you have faced in the past, being told that your child has diabetes is a major life event. All parents are devastated with the diagnosis. For the child, it is often a bit of a blur, especially as they may not be feeling well at the time.

Children remember how they were told and particular bits about what they were told. The parts that seem to stick out are about not eating sweets and having to do injections. Once those words are spoken, it is difficult to expect a child to take in anything else. It can be difficult to explain about diabetes and the need for long-term injections and blood tests. In the past, medicine may have been used to make your child feel better. Now you will need to explain why this medicine is needed forever.

Often children adapt well to getting diabetes, especially at the beginning. They may remember more about how their parents dealt with their diagnosis than how they did. For a child who is dependent on their parents, any cause for upset to their parent will upset them. Children feel more upset and scared when they know their mum or dad is upset and they don't know why. Being upset, angry and scared is a normal response. Pretending it is not there will not help you or your child. How you react to your child's diagnosis will affect how your family, friends, your child's school and ultimately your child deals with it.

There are more wrong than right ways of telling your child that diabetes has arrived in their life. It is easy to get it wrong for the right reasons, as you will be in shock too. Often what parents tell their children, they are telling themselves. Understanding how you feel about the diagnosis first would be ideal, but there is rarely time. Parents often feel impotent. It may be the first time in their child's life that they are powerless to help. It is often less distressing for the child, particularly if they are allowed to take some ownership of their diabetes. As a parent, you can never have complete ownership of your child's diabetes. You may try but this won't help them or you in the long run. Any attempt by a parent to regain control can cause a child to rebel, become irritated or be held back from managing their own diabetes and becoming independent.

I remember more about my Mum worrying about my diabetes than me...at first it was just a word...I just got on with it and did as I was told.

(Mike, 27, diagnosed aged 11)

I thought that if I had an injection I'd be all right. I didn't think I'd have to keep on injecting.

(Jason, 27, diagnosed aged 7)

I just sat there while Mum tried to take everything in. That was the start of her taking responsibility for my care all on her own...I did what I was asked to, I didn't fully understand what was going on.

(Rebecca, 35, diagnosed aged 6)

I remember going to the GP and having a blood test, then being at the hospital and having loads more tests. I had to go to the hospital every morning to do my injection. I didn't want to go to the hospital, I didn't understand why I had to go.

(Janina, 13, diagnosed aged 7)

Q **Could you suggest what I should say?**

A Here is one example of 'How to do it', which could be given to your child, a little at a time, depending on their age, stage of development and personality.

❝ When you have a temperature you don't feel well. That is because your body likes everything to be just right, not too high like when you have a temperature, and not too low, like when you're very cold and need to wear lots of jumpers. The same is true for the sugar in your blood. You need sugar in your blood for energy to run around and play games. The sugar comes from things we eat, like bread, potatoes, rice, fruit and cereal. It must not be too high or too low or you feel unwell.

With diabetes your body does not know how to stop the sugar in your blood from going too high, which is why you haven't been feeling very well. So, the doctors have to give you a medicine to bring the sugar in your blood down. If you have too much medicine your blood sugar will go too low. To get just the right amount of medicine, we will need to check how much sugar is in your blood using a small machine, smaller than a Game Boy.

When you eat it makes sugar rise in your blood. To get the right sugar level so that you feel great, the doctors will help Mummy, Daddy and you decide how much medicine you need, depending on what you eat. At the moment the only way to give the medicine, which is called insulin, is by an injection. It is not the sort of injection that you think of straight away. The needle is really small and thin so you don't feel it much, but it is still an injection. Of course no one likes having injections.

Many people have diabetes needing this type of injection and we don't know it because they get on and have fun in their lives. You will still go to school, on school trips, holidays and play games and sports. We just need to try to plan things a bit more than other people. Soon, it will be part of what we think about every day, like packing lunch for school and doing our teeth after breakfast. I wish this was something that would go away but it is something that we will need to carry on. We will all do it together with the doctors and nurses. ƨ

Q **Will my son blame me for his diabetes?**

A The issue of blame is something that comes from parents and rarely crosses the minds of children themselves, even if it does come up in arguments over unrelated things. You will want to know 'Why my child?' and this will lead on to the question of whether you are to blame.

Parents often blame themselves, even though they are told it is not their fault and even if they know deep down it isn't. It is a natural feeling to look for blame and to wish it was you and not your child who has diabetes. You may go through the same stages people go through when they are grieving the loss of someone close who has died – feeling numb, denial, anger, sadness and (hopefully sooner rather than later) acceptance. You may be grieving the loss of your child's 'perfect' life before diabetes reared its head and of a carefree childhood. Lizzie's mum in Case 1 sums it up well when she says, 'as a parent, you want your children to be perfect and have a perfect life'. However, as D W Winicott the child psychoanalyst described, health is not just the absence of disease. I take this to mean that your child's health is made up not just of physical but also emotional elements.

For a child with diabetes, understanding why their parent is upset can be confusing. Is it all because of their diabetes, they may wonder, which may make a child worry that they are to blame for their parent's sadness. It may then make it harder for a child to open up and they may feel a need to 'be strong' for you. Then you may not talk as it's too upsetting and the difficult situation just gets worse. So, now you are both all clammed up and everyone is upset.

Just as you will want to know 'Why him?', children will also want to know 'Why me?', especially when it sinks in that diabetes is forever and they are never allowed a day off. 'Why me?' is not the same as 'I blame you'.

Diabetes is full of myths, some of which your child may be told by well-meaning but ill-informed people. It may make your child attribute blame incorrectly, just as George did (see below). This was something that bothered him until he talked to me for the purposes of this book, aged 35.

Mum thinks I have diabetes because she had it when she was pregnant with me. Sometimes she cries and says she wishes it were her that has diabetes and not me.

(Mai, 8, diagnosed aged 7)

I thought it was my Mum's fault because she gave me too many sweets. It made me feel angry.

(George, 35, diagnosed aged 9)

Mum always says she wishes she could take it [diabetes] away from me. She thinks that 'cos sometimes she does my injection and it hurts and she thinks that she's hurting me. I think it's silly for parents to feel guilty.

(Kaya, 12, diagnosed aged 10)

Mum lost two stone when I was in hospital.

(Mike, 27, diagnosed aged 11)

Q Tania seemed to adapt really well when she was first diagnosed. Now she's moody and goes quiet all the time. What can I do?

A Many children adapt well initially to their diabetes. Learning the routines can be a novelty; although for some, the regular injections and being told what you are 'allowed' and 'not allowed' to eat can be overwhelming or just irritating. When the novelty of presents, fuss and new routines wears off the reality hits in that diabetes is forever. Realising that you cannot miss an injection and that you are expected to follow a 'diabetic diet', even though that may not be what it is called, day in and day out, is when the impact of diagnosis really starts to set in. It seems like, and is, forever. Especially for children diagnosed when very young, there can be a distressing time, at about 10 or 11 years, when they realise it is forever.

It's not surprising that children, and adults, have blips, lash out or

continued on next page

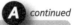

continued

become sad. Some children may seem to be 'coping wonderfully' but maybe this is not a normal response to having to do blood tests, injections and live a restricted lifestyle. Could Tania be putting on a brave face?

The time when a child realises that diabetes is for ever is a time bomb with a variable fuse. It may be a slow process. It may be a sudden realisation in response to something someone says to them, even if unintentional.

Many children just seem to get on with the diabetes routine of blood tests, injections, food balancing and hypos. At some point, however, many get fed up, particularly if an aspect of the diabetes happens at an inconvenient time or something else is going on.

Often children do not talk about their feelings but act them out in other ways, like Aiden, below. Your child may feel hassled with the constant reminders of the rules of what to eat, when to do a blood test and injection time. There may not be time to talk about how they are feeling. They may not be able to talk about it with you. Don't take this personally. It may be because you are the person who has to do the reminding. Young children are not able to answer 'Why?' questions which require a more adult thought pattern. You may need to find other ways of exploring how they feel.

For you, diabetes may be present all the time. However, for your child, they may only remember and think of their diabetes at blood test or injection time or if they have a hypo. Some children can feel alone and isolated and that no one understands how they feel. If you do not have diabetes, it is true that you will not be able to understand how they are feeling, just as they will never fully understand how you must be feeling as a parent.

I hate being diabetic...it slows down and interrupts your life. ...Sometimes I write DIABETES in big letters on a piece of paper and then punch it.

(*Aiden, 9, diagnosed aged 4*)

It didn't bother me at first...it was part of something to do and finding time to do it...it became a problem later...I became angry that my brother wasn't diabetic...that I was the only one that had to do blood tests, injections and eat an extra snack.

(George, 35, diagnosed aged 9)

Q Sam gets really annoyed when I ask him if he feels OK. I know it must be irritating, but I can't help it – I worry about him all the time. I just can't seem to say anything right.

A Well, wouldn't you get annoyed too if you were asked if you were OK all the time? No one likes being asked over and again if they are all right, especially when they are not. Your child, just like Sam, will be feeling 'normal' most of the time. By talking constantly about diabetes you really will make him feel like 'a diabetic'. Children only feel 'diabetic' when their blood is low or very high, when they're doing a blood test or an injection, or when they are asked about it.

Worrying continuously will be irritating and may make Sam start worrying, rather than getting on with his everyday life. Being overprotective will only make him feel more different. It may also stop Sam from being independent and doing what other children of his age are doing.

Living with diabetes can feel like an uphill task. Some children can't or don't share their feelings. Sometimes it may be because they think there is no point. After all, who could understand if they don't have it? Then the continual demands to do blood tests, injections, think about hypos, football and homework. It would be a lot for anyone to deal with.

The younger the child, the less likely they are to be able to answer the adult question of 'Why?' Trying to find out what is going on without asking sounds difficult but often leads to an answer. Drawing pictures can be a big clue to real feelings. Just talking about a situation that has happened and listening to the answer may also be revealing.

continued on next page

continued

At some point your child is going to need to leave home, live independently and do their own thing. Letting your child take an active part as soon as possible, even if it does result in a few mistakes, is going to make your child feel that you trust them. 'As soon as possible' must be at the right time for them. This may not be the right time for you. Pushing a child into taking things over too early can be as damaging as remaining too controlling and assuming you know everything about what your child feels. We don't expect children to cook, shop or do their laundry, so why should they do their own diabetes care if they don't want to? Ultimately you will know your child best and will need to trust your instincts but also allow some guidance from your diabetes team who will have a good general knowledge and experience base to draw upon.

People are always asking me 'Are you alright? It's so annoying.

(Lizzie, 27, diagnosed aged 8)

Mum always rings me up and the first thing she asks is 'What's your blood sugar?' I think, why doesn't she ask me 'How are you?', instead of 'Why's your blood high or low?', and 'What are you going to do about it?' It really pisses me off.

(Juliet, 22, diagnosed aged 17)

I like it when people ask me about diabetes, I can explain it to them. I say I have to balance my food and my insulin.

(Luke, 17, diagnosed aged 15)

Mum and Dad thought very differently about my diabetes. Mum felt so guilty and felt my life would be made easier if she took it all over from me. It was the burden she wanted to take away. But it was very controlling.

(Ruth, 38, diagnosed aged 14)

Q **'Diabetic' or 'person with diabetes'?**

A Some children with diabetes like to be called a diabetic whilst others hate it.

For the many children with diabetes who do not know anyone else in the same position as them, being 'a diabetic' gives them a sense of identity. Children with diabetes can feel alone, even if their family is worrying or looking after them all the time. In fact, this can increase a child's isolation and make them feel different to other children and from the rest of their family. At least if they are a 'diabetic' they know who they are. It explains to them and those around them why they have to do this and that, in PE, and at friends' parties.

For others, being labelled as 'the diabetic' is negative, just highlighting that they are different. No child wants to be different, unless it is because they won a medal at Sports Day. Being a 'diabetic' is a reminder of injections, blood tests, hospitals and not eating sweets whenever they want. Labelling all children with diabetes as 'diabetic' implies that they are all the same, with the same feelings and needing the same treatment. It also reinforces the idea that their life should fit in around their diabetes, rather than their diabetes fitting in with their life.

Being a 'diabetic' makes those less clued up about diabetes make assumptions. How many times will a non-diabetic declare, 'You're not allowed to eat that'. Not only is this annoying but it encourages the idea that all diabetics are destined for the same outcome and must live by the same rules in the Diabetic Do and Don't Rulebook.

It doesn't bother me at all. I don't know why people get so het up about it. It doesn't affect how people see you. People's perception of you is the most important thing and that's not necessarily the same as how you are referred to.

(Nigel, 37, diagnosed aged 3)

If people see my Medic Alert bracelet and ask 'Are you diabetic?' I just answer, 'I'll tell you if you tell me what colour underwear you're wearing.'

(Lizzie, 27, diagnosed aged 8)

I'm a person with diabetes....not all diabetics are the same.

(George, 35, diagnosed aged 9)

I'm diabetic. I do have diabetes and it is part of who I am. To say 'I have diabetes' is passive as if it's been given to me and I'm not in control of it. I'm diabetic – it's an active way of looking at it.

(Katherine, 30, diagnosed aged 9)

I hate the word 'chronic illness'– it makes you feel like you're on your death bed.

(Mike, 27, diagnosed aged 11)

What you can do

Here are some general suggestions about what you could focus on and certain things to avoid. However, it isn't a strict recipe, as your child is unique and special. What you say and how you say it will depend on your child's age, developmental level and personality. You will need to tailor what you say to your child. After all, you know them best.

- **Get support** right from the start. Contact Juvenile Diabetes Research Foundation (www.jdrf.org.uk) for a KIDSAC pack. It provides easy-to-digest information and support at the time of diagnosis, and helpful materials for your child, including Rufus the Bear with Type 1 Diabetes. JDRF also has useful literature; see the Appendix.

- **Remember that you know your child best, but your diabetes team has a broad level of experience and lots of knowledge.** The combination of the two make for a powerful team and neither can manage without the other.

- **Give yourself some time** to let it sink in as well as to deal with the information overload. There is time to absorb information in chunks.

- **Be there for children to answer their questions in their own time.** You may not know a lot of the answers to begin with, so you could write them down and bring them to your next meeting with your diabetes team. It will also help acknowledge to your child that you take their questions and concerns seriously.

- **Try not to make light of it, but at the same time don't lay it on too thickly** or you may cause it all to be scary and confusing.

- **Try and avoid diabetes clichés** such as 'Now you have diabetes you are not allowed to eat sweets'.

- **Share each other's memories** and see how they differ. This may help when you realise you are nagging or they accuse you of it!

- **Try not to pretend to yourself or your child** that diabetes is ever anything other than an inconvenience, or you will not be telling the whole truth. If you pretend to your child that you are not upset your child will know that you are feeling sad and maybe not understand why. You will need to explain to them without this adding to their emotional burden.

- **Never say that a cure is just around the corner.** Research developments are difficult to predict. It also suggests that life is not worth living until then, which is not the case.

- **Find a pocket of time for yourself** in all the business around diagnosis and the early stages.

Rachel's view

I have always hated being labelled as a diabetic, especially by the medical profession. It's lazy and means that doctors are not using their brains to think about me as an individual person and tailor treatment accordingly. I'm Rachel and I also have diabetes, not 'Rachel the diabetic'. If I am asked, 'How long have you been diabetic?' I answer, 'If you are asking how long I have had diabetes, then I will answer your question: 23 years'. No one gets away with that twice.

It seems to me that diagnosis is worse mostly for parents. Lies, or rather false truths since they are uninformed bits of information, are told to children from the beginning by those who are not clued up. This can be anybody, including family friends or medics. Imagine being told you can never eat sweets. What a thing to say to a 7-year-old! No wonder that produces tears. Certainly, diabetes is a lot to take on board but nothing stops you from going out there and grabbing life except for fear and poor diabetes control. The poor control may come from neglect, stemming from fear, denial or rebellion, or from lack of knowledge. Your child may have erratic blood glucose levels because their regimen does not suit them. You and your diabetes team need to find a regimen that fits your child, not try to fit the child to the regimen. Throw blame in the bin. Scaring children and their parents really upsets me. It's time to get on with life.

Many people say that there are worse things to have than diabetes. I don't find this useful as it belittles an individual's own feelings about having diabetes and can even make you feel guilty for having those feelings.

I am frustrated by the poor start that some children with diabetes have. Good diabetes care comes from routine and stability. If children are not given this, chances are their diabetes will always be hard to control. To me, this is the biggest injustice, far bigger than a diagnosis of diabetes on its own. Well-adjusted children often come from well-adjusted parents. For those who are not given such a start, this is an unfair disadvantage.

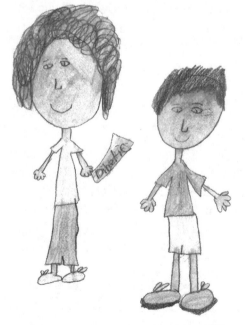

This drawing of Rachel and a young boy with diabetes was made by his sister. It was teasing Rachel as it shows her with a label attached saying 'diabetic'.

2

Hypoglycaemia

What is hypoglycaemia?

Hypoglycaemia occurs when the blood glucose levels are below the normal range, around 5 mmol/l. In those without diabetes, the body starts to react to prevent the blood glucose dropping further at levels of around 3.6–3.9 mmol/l. In those with diabetes, hypoglycaemia is defined as a blood glucose below 4.0 mmol/l and this is when you and your child will need to act. An easy way to remember this is 'Four is the floor'. In 'mild' hypoglycaemia the person can treat themselves; in 'moderate' hypoglycaemia they will need someone else to help treat their hypo. In 'severe' hypoglycaemia they may be unconscious or only partly conscious. Someone needs to give an injection of the hormone glucagon to raise the blood glucose.

Some children may feel that their blood glucose level is low when it is normal or even high if their body, more specifically their brain, has become used to running at higher levels.

What are the causes of hypoglycaemia?

Hypoglycaemia results from an imbalance between insulin, food and exercise. Too much insulin or exercise in proportion to too little glucose-containing food will cause hypoglycaemia (hypo). Exercise such as sport can cause hypos up to 1–2 days later. Your diabetes team will help find ways of dealing with exercise that suits your child, such as by eating a snack before exercise and/or reducing the insulin dose. Exercise is discussed in more detail in Chapter 3.

The symptoms of hypoglycaemia arise for two reasons. The first is the effect of the body's response to stop or reverse the hypo from happening. Hormones, the body's chemical messengers, are released into the bloodstream to try to raise the blood glucose. This is called a counter-regulatory response and in those without diabetes, would normally cause symptoms at a blood glucose level of around 3.0 mmol/l. However, in those with diabetes, this will depend on what the blood glucose normally runs at, any recent low or high blood glucose, exercise, sleep and age. The first hormone released is adrenaline; this produces symptoms such as a fast pounding pulse rate, feeling shaky, sick and sweaty. Adrenaline is normally released to allow the body to respond well to stress – that is why the early hypo symptoms may feel like stress or anxiety. The hormone glucagon is also released to cause a more sustained rise in blood glucose. Glucagon works by breaking down glycogen stores from the liver. This makes people more prone to hypos during the day after a severe hypo as the glycogen stores may be empty.

Parents of children with Type 1 diabetes are given supplies of an artificial form of the hormone glucagon for emergency use (see p. 30). The other cause of hypo symptoms is due to the direct effect of low blood glucose in the brain. In those without diabetes these effects tend to occur at a blood glucose level of around 2.5 mmol/l. The brain, like any other part of the body, needs glucose as an energy supply and if blood glucose levels are low the brain will not work properly. This may cause difficulty in concentrating and hearing, headaches, confusion, drowsiness, blurred vision and slurred speech. The body will try to stop the fall in blood glucose but if the levels are dangerously low and a hypo is untreated a person with diabetes may fall unconscious and even have a fit.

Hypoglycaemia unawareness

If someone runs low blood glucose levels a lot of the time the body may think this is normal for them. They may not then get any warning that they are having a hypo from the effect of the hormones that are realeased to counteract the hypo. This is called 'hypoglycaemia unawareness' and can be dangerous as the person may not know they are hypo and, if their blood glucose falls too low, they may fall unconscious. This is reversible by avoiding hypoglycaemia completely for 2–3 weeks.

How can you tell someone is having a hypo?

How someone looks or feels can also be explained by the body's response to hypoglycaemia. As the body tries to bring up the blood sugar your child may be irritable, behaving unusually for them, looking pale, sweaty and trembly. You may notice that they are confused or have slurred speech.

What is the best way to treat a hypo?

The severity of the hypo, your child's age, the type of insulin your child is on, and recent exercise are just some of the factors that will determine how to treat the hypo. The insulin regimen may also explain what time of day they tend to go hypo, although this will also depend on food intake, exercise and injection sites.

In mild and moderate hypoglycaemia, children need a fast-acting sugar, such as glucose tablets. They could have Lucozade, coke or orange juice if they prefer. You will need to wait up to 10–15 minutes before you see the blood glucose start to rise. You may need to give more glucose after this point if the blood glucose hasn't started to rise. Glucose or a sugary drink is preferred to foods such as chocolate and cake which are sweet but fatty, because fat causes glucose to get into the blood less quickly than glucose on its own. This means that the hypo will not be reversed as quickly. Except for those on insulin pumps, who can lower the basal insulin rate, children usually also need a longer-acting starchy food, such as a cereal bar, to stop another hypo happening later.

Children having a hypo may be awake but unable to chew glucose tablets or take a sweet drink. If they can swallow, glucose gels are useful and practical. If your child is not awake or is having a fit, you will need to give them an injection of glucagon into a muscle. It comes in an orange-coloured box, and is given by injection into muscle when a child has a severe hypo and is unconscious, as discussed below. Your diabetes team will show you how to do this. You will need, and probably want, to go to hospital if this occurs. If your child is unconscious, it is important not to give anything by mouth, including glucose gel, because of the risk of choking.

Glucagon can make people feel sick and even vomit, sometimes only after 1–2 hours. Sometimes the glucagon injection does not work to raise the blood glucose. This can happen if the liver's glycogen stores are already depleted, having already been broken down to produce glucose to counteract a hypo during the previous day, or after extreme exercise. If

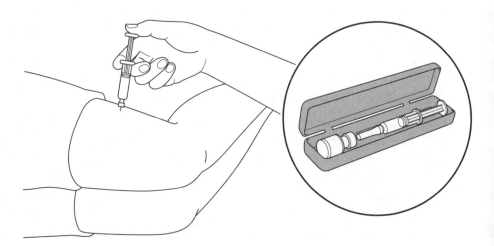

Injecting glucagon into muscle

this happens, you will need to call an ambulance or go to hospital immediately for intravenous glucose.

It is important not to overtreat hypos, although this is easier said than done because witnessing and experiencing hypos can be frightening. Overtreating hypos occurs frequently, as you feel like eating until your symptoms start to go away, and should not be underestimated. It is worth being clear about your child's hypo treatment with your diabetes team as overtreatment will cause a rapid swing to high blood glucose.

Will hypos cause long-term damage?

Having hypos will affect an individual's ability to concentrate and perform tasks. Most of the effects disappear within minutes. However, with more severe hypos the effects may last up to 24 hours. Mild to moderate hypos will not cause any long-term damage. It is still unclear whether severe and sustained hypos causing unconsciousness may affect brain functioning in the long term. As most brain development occurs in the first five years of life, in particular the first two years of life, it is best if severe hypos are avoided in this age group, although sometimes this is easier said than done.

Will they wake up if they have a hypo at night?

Night-time hypos are often a parent's biggest fear. Most children will either wake up if they have a night-time hypo or sleep through it and still be all right in the morning. Others may have nightmares or complain of headaches or feeling tired on waking. A hypo at night may cause a blood glucose reading to be high in the morning because normal stress hormones have been released to raise the blood glucose to counteract the hypo. This is called the **rebound phenomenon**. Even if a child has a hypo severe enough to fit, usually this will stop on its own. Diabetic keto-acidosis, due to skipping insulin injections, is a more likely cause of death in diabetes than hypoglycaemia.

I am often asked about the 'Dead-in-Bed' syndrome, the sudden death at night of someone with diabetes. I cannot stress enough how *extremely rare* this is. It is not often discussed in clinic but is a frequent cause of worry and distress for parents. The cause of the syndrome is not known, making it difficult to advise about prevention. Some theories about cause include hypoglycaemia at night causing an arrhythmia (heart rhythm disturbance). Such a hypo may have occurred because of taking the wrong type or amount of evening insulin.

This fear needs to be kept in balance; avoiding hypos at night is important but so is avoiding marked hyperglycaemia. If you are worried about night hypos there are several things you can do.

■ Test your child's blood glucose before bed. You could also test occasionally in the night, such as when you get in from a late night out. You could also ask your diabetes clinic if they have a continuous glucose monitor (CGM), to measure the glucose at night over a few days, as described in more detail in Chapter 3.

■ Give your child a snack before bed. This advice may depend on the insulin regimen, so discuss this with your diabetes team. Discuss changing the insulin regimen if it is not working for your child.

■ Discuss with your diabetes team what bedtime glucose to aim for. Your doctor may advise that you should try to keep the blood glucose at bedtime slightly higher than at other times, depending on the type of insulin your child is on.

Case 1

Paint me a hypo

On a summer camp for young people with diabetes, children were asked to paint a hypo. They were better able to put their thoughts into pictures. In the poem below I imagined what the children were trying to express in their drawings. Each stanza is about one drawing.

Man trapped in a Caged Cell
Stuck in the mud of a shadow
Somehow dodging the glare
　　through the bars from
The Other Side.

Jekyll and Hyde
A switch to
The Other Me
Which I see as One
Each snippet of time.

People dissolving
Smaller
Smaller
Floating up,
Those helium-filled people,
As my head begins to spin and
My BMs drop.

A column of blood is all I am
Blood which may be
High
Low
Sometimes just right.

Invisible brain
Whose pandemonium is
Inexplicable to those
Outside
My trembling head.

A wobbly smile or
Half-misunderstood frown
Tears trickle down my now pale
cheeks.

As for me?
I can be all of these and have
been
But still I am me.

Originally published in
Diabetic Medicine,
Blackwell 2002; 19:343

Seeing her fighting and hitting me when low and refusing juice is stressful.

(A mum describes the stress of witnessing a hypo)

Discussion

Hypos can be frightening to experience as well as to witness. The poem above and the picture (on p. 39) explaining how children feel when having a hypo may surprise and upset you. Pictures can capture a lot more than the words can express. They show how scary a hypo can feel.

Although all the experiences are different, the common themes may explain why your child behaves in a certain way – being upset, irritable, agitated, scared or not being 'there'. Given those feelings, it would be easy to understand why some prefer to run their blood glucose a bit higher just to avoid having a hypo or avoid hypos at all costs. For others, having a mild hypo is no big deal and a great reason to eat some sweets. Some people tell me they enjoy hypos, but perhaps it is the treatment they enjoy.

Having hypos is part of having diabetes. Some hypos are avoidable by understanding a child's own routine. Others will just happen and often without a good explanation. Having no hypos at all may mean that your child's blood glucose levels are running high a lot of the time, which can bring its own problems (see Chapter 6: Hyperglycaemia, ketoacidosis and complications). The opposite is also true – having too many hypos is also not a good thing, both because of the inconvenience they bring but also because severe hypos can be dangerous and may lead to the body feeling as if hypos are 'normal', resulting in lack of awareness. Whether or not having hypos with diabetes is a 'normal' or even a 'good thing', for the person who has to experience them, it can be embarrassing, inconvenient, frightening or just a darned nuisance.

Most children will remember being woken, or waking themselves, because of a hypo during the night. It can be horrid – it's dark, and they are not feeling right. Some children might wake up and be confused, and wander about for a bit getting more confused. Being tired or having more hypos the next day can feel like a punishment.

Young children often do not recognise when they are hypo. You will learn how to recognise hypos for them. This will be particular to each individual. It may be because of a change in their behaviour, such as becoming quiet, more active or aggressive, or a change in their appearance, such as becoming pale or sweaty.

Ultimately your child will need in time to learn about their own hypos and how to recognise and treat them themselves, in order to lead an independent life.

Case 2

Hypo memories

Introducing Jeffrey, 9, diagnosed aged 4

Sometimes I have bad dreams that something bad has happened. I take too much insulin and then I'm in hospital.

When you're hypo your belly hurts and you're sweating a bit. If you take [eat] something it takes a while. Your belly still hurts so you think it's not working so you take a bit more [food]. But then you do your sugar level and it's high.

If you have a hypo in front of other people they might crowd around you – too many voices.

I kind of feel a bit bad and a bit funny. When I was 7 I wasn't sure what it felt like. I started to get the idea when I was 8.

Discussion

Jeffrey describes the fear experienced when having a hypo. He has been hospitalised before due to a severe hypo and carries this memory with him. He also describes his experiences of a hypo and why it is easy for those with diabetes, as well as for those treating hypos, to overtreat them. It is easy to give advice about waiting some minutes before seeing the effect of the hypo reversed with treatment. In practice, it is easier said than done. For your child who is experiencing the hypo, they just want it to go away. Witnessing hypos can also be frightening and you may want to give your child more and more food to get them out of it. However, they may then go high later just because of overtreating the hypo rather than due to rebound (see p. 31). It is important not to treat any rebound with extra insulin otherwise your child may go into another hypo and blood glucose will be rising and falling so unpredictably that you won't know where you are. You will work out what's best with a little trial and error.

The other issue Jeffrey raises is that when he is having a hypo people crowd around him. There are 'too many voices'. Many of us who have hypos do not like people talking to us. It is too much to cope with whilst having a hypo. Even worse than talking, is when people talk loudly: they do it because they are afraid. People tend to ask others they see in distress, loudly, 'ARE YOU ALL RIGHT?' Generally, we want to be left quietly and not talked to whilst we eat our glucose until we start to feel better. My advice would be to sit quietly next to your child offering them their hypo treatment and waiting for them to initiate conversation. Of course this will not apply to very young children who often do not recognise what is going on.

Case 3

Different types of hypos

Introducing Jason, 27, diagnosed aged 7

I often mistreat a hypo and eat too much. It's a survival instinct – your body tells you that you need to eat, you open the fridge and gorge. Something makes you feel really hungry.

There are different types of hypos. I feel really tired and sleepy. Then I realise I'm hypo and I'm back to my normal self. Self-doubt. I'm trying to do something and I start questioning everything. I feel really strange. You're falling into a hypo but you're not thinking. So you can overlook that you're having a hypo.

It can be dangerous. Sometimes at night I can't sleep worrying about things irrationally. Suddenly I realise that I'm having a hypo. Hollow, something's missing and you want to curl up into a ball. Other times, my brain can function well but I lose control of my limbs and actions. I can see where I want to go but I'm falling over, like when I did my injection and was watching the cricket on television, which is a really slow game. Suddenly I realised I was hypo and I was trying to get to the garage to get the Lucozade. My brain knew where I wanted to get to but I couldn't get there. Once I started fighting people when out playing golf with friends and then collapsed. It was the first time my friends had seen me like that.

Discussion

Even though Jason is an adult, he admits to still overtreating hypos. He is aware that he does it but he still tends to overtreat them. It highlights really well the instinctual feeling that a hypo brings and the feeling of needing to get your blood glucose level up up *up*, now now *now*.

It is easy to overreact to a hypo, both by the person having the hypo and the person treating it. Many people feel a 'hunger rage' and want to devour everything in their sight. As the body's natural defence reactions to having a hypo will also kick in, overtreating the hypo in combination with this effect may cause high blood glucose hours later (see rebound phenomenon on p. 31). The hunger is not a real hunger, but a desire and urgent need for food.

With some discussion, thought and planning, it is possible to make a decision not to overtreat hypos. If you think you or your child are prone to overtreating hypos it would be worth asking your diabetes team to remind you how much is needed to treat a hypo. This will depend on the age of your child.

Jason also describes how he can have different types of hypos. This may depend on other distracting things that are going on, or the rate of fall of the blood glucose level. A slow fall in blood glucose can cause a sudden realisation of already being in a hypo. If the blood glucose falls rapidly it can also be really sudden and make you feel off-kilter. Some of us may feel hypo just because the blood glucose is falling rapidly even if you check the level and it is normal. Many also confuse the symptoms of being low and high, so it is always worth doing a blood test to confirm a hypo before starting treatment. If your child thinks they are having a hypo in this situation, sit them down and recheck their blood glucose again in a few minutes. Your child will often be correct and they are now having a hypo, rather than just wanting some sweets.

Case 4

Hypo fear
Introducing Daniel, 17, diagnosed aged 12

Sometimes I forget or miss my injection. At the beginning I was told to give 30 units of long-acting [insulin] at night. It was too much, I kept having hypos and getting up in the night and not sleeping.

Before I didn't know how to adjust my insulin so I stopped taking it for several months and just took fast-acting.

It was mostly a deliberate thing so I didn't ever go into a hypo. For me, when I'm hypo I feel weak. If I don't eat something now I'm going to fall and go to sleep. I feel safer if I'm a bit higher and not too low. If you're too low it's too drastic.

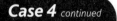

Case 4 *continued*

One time I had given my injection but I didn't feel like eating. That time I was out of it. They phoned my diabetes specialist nurses who told Mum to give me sugar in hot water. I remember waking up and being given lots of sweet drinks. I didn't feel like eating and drinking.

Discussion

Daniel has such big hypo fear that he doesn't feel he has time to test his blood glucose level to confirm he is hypo. However, he may not be. Daniel did tell me about one or two major hypos that he had in the past. He may now be having symptoms of anxiety, which can mimic hypos. Alternatively, following on from these big hypos he decided to run his blood glucose levels high to avoid having them. As a result his body may have adjusted to a higher blood glucose level and 'think it is normal' for him to experience blood glucose at a higher level. He then may experience hypo symptoms at a blood glucose level which is not low. Doing a blood test is the only way of confirming whether your child is having a hypo or not. There is usually time, except in the rare circumstance that they are not fully awake. It will also allow you and them to learn at what blood glucose level they feel hypo. This may change with time depending on their awareness, which may change with age, as well as the blood glucose levels that they are running at the time.

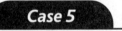

Case 5

Learning from mistakes

Introducing Mike, 27, diagnosed aged 11

I used to play the violin at school. When I was 17 it was my first time leading the school orchestra. I came on stage and did my bow. I played the first note and knew that I was low. I didn't know what to do. I couldn't just walk off stage and I didn't have any Dextrose in my pockets. I carried on but by the interval I was pouring with sweat and I had played the first half of the concert really badly. I sorted myself out in the interval and played a good second half. At the end I told the conductor I had had

continued on next page

Case 4 *continued*

a hypo and he said, 'I thought you weren't on form'!

Hypos always happen at the wrong time – the only time you need a good sleep you wake up at 2 a.m. having a hypo or if you're in a rush.

It taught me a good lesson, to test before I do anything important.

Discussion

Mike learnt two valuable lessons: to always do a blood test before doing anything important and to always carry glucose tablets with him. As Mike is now an adult and one who drives, this has stood him in good stead as he knows the importance of checking his blood glucose before he gets behind the wheel of a car and always has something to treat a hypo if he does have one when driving.

Daniel in the previous case also learned the hard way that giving insulin and not eating results in an unwanted hypo. There's a lot to be said from learning from one's own mistakes. However, for Daniel the experience of the hypo made him want to avoid another one at all costs. This is a bit extreme and in most cases children will learn that they need to eat after injecting, what they need to treat their hypo and what to do. Most know they need to sit and be still and let their blood glucose come up before rushing around again.

Most modern insulins may allow you to do the injection during or even after a meal. However, for those on two injections a day, this may not be possible. You may find yourself trying to force your child to eat to avoid a hypo. This can become an ongoing battle. It can be particularly difficult to persuade young children to eat when they don't want to. Speak with your diabetes team if this is your problem, as your child may benefit from changing insulin regimen, such as to a basal bolus regimen or an insulin pump (see Chapter 4).

However, for young children or those who are 'fussy eaters' discuss this with your diabetes team: it may be possible to inject after you have seen what they have eaten. This works well on a basal bolus regimen (see Chapter 4). Even if your child hasn't eaten anything they will still need some insulin on board. If they are on a long-acting insulin injection lasting 24 hours, this might be enough without any short-acting if they haven't eaten. You will need to discuss this scenario with your diabetes team.

Q What does it feel like to have a hypo?

A If you ask ten people with diabetes what it feels like to have a hypo, you are likely to get ten different answers. There are symptoms common to hypos, such as feeling wobbly, shaky, vacant, hungry and sweaty; tiredness, a racing heart; feeling sick and having blurry vision. Even though some of those feelings may be similar, in each person with diabetes those feelings in their body will be different. Feeling wobbly to one person may be like floating up like a balloon, but to another like trying to balance on an inflatable raft on a rough sea. Some also find it hard to differentiate between being high and low.

Many young people get cross when those without diabetes say they know what a hypo feels like, thinking its like when they have missed a meal or feel hungry. Few people without diabetes experience hypos because the body is able to regulate their blood glucose instantly and stop it dropping too low.

You will only come close to knowing what your child feels like when they have a hypo if you ask them. The words that children use may only touch the surface of how it makes them feel. Drawing pictures is one way of allowing, in particular, young children, to express their feelings.

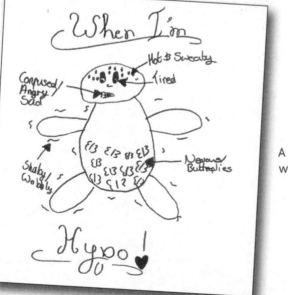

A girl aged 12 drew what it feels like to be hypo.

39

My hair goes funny when I have a hypo...I look in the mirror to check.

(Darren, 12)

Everything slows down and goes blurry....fast and slow at the same time.

(Luke, 17)

Hypos are quite annoying. If you're in the middle of something you have to do your blood test.

(Margaret, 12)

I don't like the feeling when I'm hypo. I go shaky and feel irritated. Mum overdoses me on sugar. I guess she's scared of hypos too.

(Janina, 13)

Having a hypo is a bit like being drunk without the fun part. I feel shaky, wobbly and nauseous.

(Katherine, 30)

I go dizzy and hazy, like in a movie when everything's all fast at different times.

(Summer, 13)

My speech becomes more confused. I'm in the middle of a sentence and I can't remember what I'm saying. My brain short cuts. I can't keep hold of anything in my head and there's dizziness between my eyes.

(Ruth, 38)

● *Low*	● *Sick*
● *Wobbly*	● *I'm starved*
● *Feel hypo*	● *Pins and needles*
● *Tired*	● *Feel funny*
● *Tummy hurts/ tummy ache*	● *Poorly*
● *Shaky*	● *Dizzy*
● *Weak*	● *Sweaty*
● *Hungry*	● *Headache*

Children use these words to describe having a hypo

Q Earl tries to avoid hypos, especially at school, by overeating or refusing to give more insulin. What should I do?

A It depends on why Earl is avoiding them. Has he had a bad hypo in the past? Does he want to avoid unnecessary attention at school? Is he trying to fit in with the crowd? There will be a reason and finding it may be part of the solution. Speak with your diabetes team: maybe a change in insulin regimen may be a solution, or more support, or just talking things through with others who understand. Once the reason is found, Earl may be able to help find the answer himself, with your help and that of the diabetes team.

If you have a hypo at school people just see you eating sweets. Then they want to eat some.
(Kaya, 12)

Once I fainted because of a bad hypo in school. When I came round I was on the floor and a boy in my class said 'I think George is on drugs'.
(George, 35)

I used to be scared of hypos and keep my levels high.
(Luke, 17)

Q Katie doesn't always recognise that she is having a hypo. I can tell, even before she knows. If I suggest she checks her blood sugar she gets really angry and just refuses to do it. Often I have to wait until she is almost collapsing and then force her to eat something. Have you any suggestions?

A It can be most annoying to be told to do something. If your child is having a hypo and refusing to let you do a blood test or eat anything, you will likely feel a mixture of fear, frustration and anxiety.

A child's refusal to check their blood sugar and treat a hypo and

continued on next page

A *continued*

being, in your opinion, 'blooming difficult', may be a symptom of the hypo itself. A child's behaviour may completely change when they are hypo.

If you talk to Katie when she is not having a hypo she may recognise that she becomes a bit difficult with a hypo and when you suggest checking her blood sugar she realises that she does feel a bit weird. However, some children may not even remember how they behave when they had a hypo. Many children when having a hypo hate that phrase 'Are you feeling all right?' The answer 'I'm fine!!' may mean 'No, I'm not!'

I hate it when Mum asks me ' Do you feel OK?' It's so annoying.

(Juliet, 22)

Q Ben refuses to wear his medical identity bracelet. He has started going out with friends and has had a few hypos. I worry that he may have a severe hypo and is mistakenly thought to be drunk and either ignored or arrested. How can I persuade him to wear an identity bracelet or tell his friends?

A Young people want to be the same as everyone else – same sneakers, same iPod. Some young people hate wearing an identity bracelet because it makes them feel different and it is a nametag that labels them as such.

Refusing to tell your friends you have diabetes and refusing to wear a medical identity bracelet can be a dangerous combination. However, for that young person, they have a hidden condition. They don't look any different on the outside, even if they feel it on the inside. An identity bracelet will easily uncover their secret.

The problem is that alcohol can change our sense of awareness and also reduce blood sugar levels (see Chapter 9: The teenage years). An alternative is to persuade Ben to carry an identity card in his wallet: a girl could put it in her purse. That way it is hidden away unless they are in the situation when it is needed.

Q I do Lynne's blood sugar at midnight every night because she has had a couple of really bad night hypos. I have been told not to check Lynne's blood sugar every night but I worry that she will have a hypo and not wake up. Should I be checking her blood during the night or not?

A Most children either wake up or sleep through a night hypo. You might worry that your child will die in the night, but in reality this is extremely rare. Doing blood tests now and then during the night is useful but doing it every night will only add to your anxiety and sleep deprivation. It is not a good idea to disturb your child's sleep every night. Lynne may also pick up on your anxieties and start panicking about hypos herself. Spot checks are useful, as well as doing a blood test again if they have been low before going to bed. If she is having night hypos, however, speak with your diabetes team about finding a solution: maybe she needs a bigger bedtime snack or less evening insulin, or to change to a different insulin regimen.

I remember Dad sitting by my bed in the middle of the night trying to wake me up and get me to eat something because my blood [sugar] was low. It was always a glass of orange juice followed by a jam sandwich. I didn't like eating when I wasn't hungry but I knew I had to. I always knew I had had a hypo in the night because my fingers would be sticky in the morning and there would be crumbs in the bed! I'd be tired at school next day.

(Lizzie, 27)

Q Sometimes Simon takes a bigger dose of fast-acting insulin to make himself hypo so he can eat sweets. I know having a hypo makes him feel awful, so why does he do it?

A If sweets are a 'forbidden fruit', only allowed when your child has a hypo, then this is an understandable scenario. One way of preventing this situation is not to treat hypos with sweets, but to incorporate sweets, chocolates and cakes, in moderation, into a normal balanced diet.

However, the situation may still arise when your child is 'not allowed' sweets when other children are offered them. Perhaps the sweets will be put aside for when your child is 'allowed' to eat them. When should this be? At the next hypo? With the next meal? After a bit of short-acting insulin? There are no right or wrong answers. Whatever you decide will be based on your home, family and school life.

I like having hypos because you can eat sweets.

(*Darren, 12*)

There's no point having a hypo if you can't enjoy it.

(*Lizzie, 27*)

Sometimes I think I'm going hypo but actually I'm anxious. Recently sometimes I enjoy the feeling. I think, 'Cool, I can have a chocolate bar'. I do tend to overtreat them. It's a great excuse to eat chocolate.

(*Beatrice, 31*)

Q James's diabetes team have told me to give him a short-acting sugar, such a Dextrose tablets, when he has a hypo. Is it wrong to give him sweets, as it is the only time when he is really 'allowed' to eat them?

A We all crave things we think we are not allowed. One of the many myths about having diabetes is that you are not allowed to eat sweets. This is no longer how diabetes is managed. However, eating sweets whenever you feel like it, as may happen whether you have diabetes or not, is not ideal. If you have diabetes, the body is likely not to be able to cope. (Nor is it advisable if you do not have diabetes, for other reasons such as obesity and tooth decay.) Even if you can eat sweets and take extra insulin, and incorporate sweets into your everyday food plan, the fact remains that sweet foods raise blood glucose quickly.

If sweets are a 'forbidden fruit' and hypos are treated with sweets, the risk is that it encourages your child to want a hypo in order to get hold of some.

It is a difficult situation to be in. Your child is not feeling good in their hypo. Sweets will raise their blood glucose and your child (probably) likes sweets. Surely, you may think, they deserve some kind of treat if they are going to have a hypo. Of course they do, and children often feel pleasure in experiencing hypos knowing that Mum will produce some fruit pastilles or jelly babies for them in return. However, it can start to reinforce the idea of rewarding ill health with a forbidden fruit. Although your child is able to enjoy sweets when they are having a mild hypo, with more severe hypos it can be difficult to chew sweets or glucose tablets. It may be easier and faster to drink some Lucozade, or an equivalent glucose-containing drink. Eating when you're not hungry is not enjoyable, however nice a 'treat' it is. People with diabetes would prefer to be able to eat 'treats' when those without diabetes are eating them.

Ideally, you want your child to think positively about food and incorporate sweet foods, in moderation, into their routine. Of course those who don't have diabetes should also be doing this. The

continued on next page

A *continued*

problem is that they don't. So it just makes someone with diabetes feel left out and punished. Not only are they having blood tests, injections and hypos, but they also can't eat sweets, not even when they have a hypo.

What you can do

- **Always confirm hypoglycaemia** with a blood glucose test, except in the rare situation of near or complete loss of consciousness.

- **Decide on how you are going to treat hypos** before they occur. This may depend on your child's age and how low their blood glucose level is. Ask your diabetes team for a plan so you know what to do when it happens.

- **Always carry some fast-acting sugar with you** and something to follow this up with.

- **Take hypos seriously but at the same time try not to panic.** Stop what you are doing and ask your child to stop for at least 15 minutes as it may take this long to see the blood glucose levels start to rise. Never leave them alone in case the blood glucose level carries on falling.

- **Offer your child hypo treatment quietly.** If you do speak, use a quiet voice.

- **Don't overtreat a hypo.** Allow 10–15 minutes before you can expect to see a difference. Hyperglycaemia can also make children feel unwell and causes problems in the long term.

Rachel's view

Hypos can be scary but mostly they are just annoying. They are inconvenient and require time to sort out and that doesn't fit in with my busy lifestyle. I could, and have, tried to run higher, but it's no good for me in the long run and I don't like how I feel when my bloods are high. I juggle my worries about having hypos with the fear of long-term complications. It might sound surprising, given that I have only had two hypos requiring assistance in my 23-year diabetic life, and also (touch wood) don't have any diabetic complications, reflecting my hard work at keeping my blood glucose levels pretty good over the years.

My first and only unconscious hypo when I passed out was shortly after I was diagnosed. My dad, who is a doctor, gave me extra insulin as he didn't want my blood sugars to be a bit high at any time, worrying about complications in the future. My second big hypo needing assistance was when I was a medical student and only had a few glucose tablets with me. I wasn't sure I would make it to the shop to get some Lucozade as a top-up, so embarrassingly had to ask someone to get it for me. I thought I was going to pass out and found it difficult to articulate what I wanted. I did manage to get my message across eventually. However, this one may have been more to do with anxiety symptoms, knowing I only had a few glucose tablets on me, and the worry about losing control rather than symptoms of a major hypo itself. I was too panicked at the time to do a blood test and not thinking straight. Never underestimate the fear of having hypos, or even the fear of the fear.

Of course I have had plenty of other hypos over the years but I have always had good awareness and always carry glucose tablets with me because I never want to be in a situation that I can't deal with. I would feel as if I had let myself down, not to mention the embarrassment factor. I tell parents, children and young people with diabetes about the importance of stopping what they're doing when they have a hypo, sitting down, being still and treating the hypo appropriately. However, when it comes to myself, I am pretty busy and often try to treat my hypo as I carry on walking. I think, this hypo is not going to get in my way! Sometimes I get away with it but usually I have to give into the hypo, sit down and munch on some Dextrose.

It amuses me when people without diabetes think a hypo feels like when they are hungry or their blood sugar is a little bit low because they haven't eaten. They don't know what it feels like and they can't know. Maybe it's unfair to expect them to; after all, they are trying to empathise. But why try? I would prefer them to say, 'I can't imagine what it feels like' and ask me to describe it to them.

3

Blood tests

What is a normal blood glucose level?

In someone who doesn't have diabetes, blood glucose is tightly controlled between about 4–7 mmol/l.

What blood glucose level should we aim for?

You will be given targets to aim for of around 4–8 mmol/l before meals and up to 10 mmol/l after eating and before bed. These are higher than the 'normal' values seen in those without diabetes in order to avoid severe hypoglycaemia, which may occur if you try and run your child's blood glucose levels too low. This is why someone without diabetes may have a blood glucose level of 3.8 mmol/l which is normal for them, but in someone with diabetes a glucose of less than 4 mmol/l is termed a hypo (see Chapter 2: Hypoglycaemia). 'Four is the floor'. It is also important not to run the blood glucose levels too high all of the time in order to reduce the risk of complications (see Chapter 6: Hyperglycaemia, ketoacidosis and complications).

Long periods of high blood glucose as well as severe hypoglycaemia don't feel nice, can affect brain functioning and hyperglycaemia in the longer term may cause complications. So the target blood glucose levels aim to achieve the lowest possible blood glucose without severe hypoglycaemia whilst avoiding long periods of hyperglycaemia. You will come across the term HbA_{1c}. This is short for 'glycoslylated haemoglobin' and is a value that is used as an indirect marker of blood glucose control over a period of two to three months. Generally speaking, an HbA_{1c} under 7.5% (59 mmol/mol) is recommended at present but this may need to be adjusted to avoid severe hypoglycaemia, particularly in young children. This is discussed in more detail in Chapter 6.

What affects blood glucose levels?

Insulin, and exercise in the presence of insulin, lower blood glucose levels, whilst carbohydrate-containing foods and hormones such as adrenaline, growth hormone, cortisol and glucagon, raise them. Exercise without enough insulin can raise blood glucose because of the release of adrenaline and cortisol (see the diagram on p. 52). When it comes to exercising, you will need to talk to your diabetes team about what to do to get the balance right. This will depend a bit on what type of insulin regimen your child is on and how strenuous and long the exercise will be. Usually exercise reduces blood glucose levels. However, with strenuous exercise and if there is not enough insulin available, blood glucose will rise. Exercise also makes you more prone to hypoglycaemia after stopping exercising, the night and even the day after. Adjustments may involve changing insulin dose and/or having some extra carbohydrate before or during exercise. You may also need less insulin after exercise, overnight after exercising and even the next day. This is because the liver's glycogen stores (which release glucose when needed) are used up and also the body is more sensitive to the insulin that is around. You will need advice from your diabetes team and to plan ahead for exercise. Any plan that is made is very individual and will depend on the type of exercise, how often your child is exercising and what the pre-exercise blood glucose is. Exercise deserves a special mention as it is an important topic and is discussed in more detail later.

What are the different ways to test blood glucose?

Checking blood glucose by fingerprick blood testing is the commonest way of checking the immediate blood glucose level. Ear lobes can also be used, although this can be technically more difficult. The forearms or the palm of the hand can be used for testing blood glucose using a special machine, but this can be unreliable if the blood glucose is changing rapidly. Blood tests will be unreliable if the blood is taken from sugary fingers, so wash hands that have been in contact with food. Most of the time it's enough just to ensure the skin is clean and dry. If the fingers are washed and left moist, the blood will run and it's difficult to get a blob of blood onto the test strip. The water can also dilute the blood giving an artificially low result.

It is also possible to check the glucose level in the interstitial fluid, which is the fluid around the cells of the tissues, using a sensor inserted under the skin that is attached to a box machine, or one that is part of an insulin pump. These are useful to see trends, especially at night, as they measure the glucose level every few minutes. However, there is a delay of up to 15 minutes between the result and that of the actual blood glucose level and it is also important to do fingerprick blood tests a few times a day in order to calibrate the machine.

Glucose can be detected in a urine test but only when the blood glucose is over about 10 mmol/l causing it to spill over into the urine. It is not a reliable marker of the actual blood glucose level, it just tells you that glucose in the blood has been a bit high over the previous few hours.

Before your child is seen in clinic you will probably be asked to take them to have either a fingerprick test, or a formal blood test to check the HbA_{1c}, which reflects the average blood glucose over the past 2–3 months.

How often should someone with diabetes test their blood glucose?

There are no set rules, but about four times a day is usually recommended, as well as at times when your child doesn't feel or look well. Don't forget that a blood test result only tells you about that moment in time. Tests at different times of the day give you different information. Testing before meals and before bed is the mainstay of blood testing. Testing at other times will also be important, such as during the night and 1½–2 hours after eating, as well as before and after exercise. You won't need to do all of these every day but it will be useful to do so sometimes to see the trend throughout the day. Your diabetes team should guide you as to when to do these extra blood tests but about twice a month is a good guide. Doing a blood test will give you an instant result in order to prevent hypoglycaemia and severe hyperglycaemia, especially when there are ketones, as well as to look at trends over several days in order to make changes (see Chapter 6 for discussion about Sick Day Rules). Testing after exercise will be important as the hypo effects of exercise can last up to the next day if the exercise is strenuous.

Why is exercise important if you have diabetes?

Exercise is important for everyone, for general heath and well-being. Regular exercise can provide a motivation for improved blood glucose control – no one would want a hypo during a game of football or to be hindered from running their fastest to score the winning goal. It can also provide structure and routine, the key to easier and improved diabetes management.

Managing diabetes with exercise is important not just to prevent hypos but also to optimise performance and to be able to get the most out of the exercise for all-round health.

Most people worry about exercise causing hypoglycaemia. However, blood glucose does not necessarily fall during exercise: it depends on the balance between how much insulin is around, how much glucose is needed for the working muscles and the type of exercise. There may need to be some fine tuning to get things spot on – if not, sometimes blood glucose control can worsen with exercise if appropriate adjustments are not made.

What happens to blood glucose with exercise if you don't have diabetes?

When anyone exercises, more blood flows to the working muscles. Blood glucose is taken up and levels start to fall. Stored glucose in the muscle (glycogen) is being used as energy. In someone without diabetes, hypoglycaemia is prevented because insulin secretion decreases and other 'counter-regulatory' hormones (glucagon, adrenaline and cortisol), which raise blood glucose, increase. Adrenaline and cortisol are 'stress hormones' and are released during exercise. Glucagon is a hormone secreted when blood glucose falls. Adrenaline, cortisol and glucagon all mobilise glucose to provide energy for exercise. Stored glucose in the liver (glycogen) is broken down to glucose to prevent hypoglycaemia. This is why endurance athletes stock up on carbohydrates before a race to fill up their glycogen stores.

What happens when someone exercises if they have Type 1 diabetes?

As someone with Type 1 diabetes has none of his or her own insulin, after the insulin has been injected it cannot be changed. Additionally, the production of the counter-regulatory hormones, which would normally raise blood glucose during exercise, may not be so swift. Both of these situations make someone with diabetes prone to hypoglycaemia.

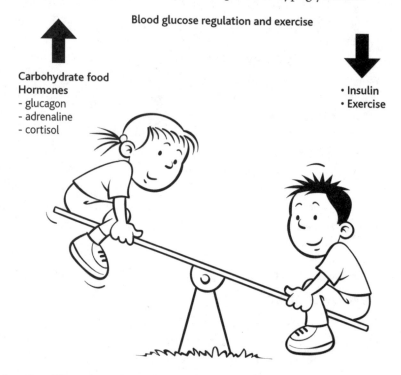

Blood glucose regulation and exercise

Carbohydrate food
Hormones
- glucagon
- adrenaline
- cortisol

• **Insulin**
• **Exercise**

Exercise affects the way blood sugar is balanced. Exercise can only lower blood glucose in the presence of insulin because with exercise other 'counter-regulatory' hormones are produced.

Without enough insulin around, blood glucose starts to rise with strenuous exercise – the type that is so intense it can only be kept up for a short period because the muscles start to hurt due to the build up of lactic acid. This can cause problems with hyperglycaemia and even ketones being produced. However, knowing about this can also be useful to prevent hypoglycaemia. For example, in sports involving bursts of strenuous exercise, such as a football game, the intense bursts may prevent the natural fall in blood glucose that might come from more gentle exercise in between those sprints. The flip side in these situations is that there may be a fall in blood glucose later, which is where having a snack comes in to refill those glycogen stores and prevent hypos. Many younger children naturally do this kind of play anyway, with periods of running and then more gentle play, but as children become older, usually from the teenage years, any exercise is usually more persistent and can be planned.

That is how it works in theory, but how an individual will react to exercise will depend on a number of factors that need to be taken into account when deciding on an individual plan of action for exercise. Adjusting insulin and snacks is necessary and is relatively straightforward, but it can only be done with blood glucose testing to know how to interpret the results and make any necessary adjustments.

Managing exercise in practice

Insulin

- **Insulin regimen**   Depending on what type of insulin your child is on, this will influence how you manage exercise, by deciding to reduce the insulin and/or take extra carbohydrate.
- **Timing of the insulin injection**   The timing in relation to exercise will determine when the fall in glucose is likely to happen. If this coincides with exercise, hypos are more likely. The opposite is also true: sport before an evening injection on a twice-a-day regimen may mean there is not a lot of insulin around and blood glucose may rise (see figure on p.55).
- **Insulin dose**   This may need to be adjusted to prevent hypos and hypers.
- **Injection site**   Injecting into the site that will be exercised results in the insulin being absorbed more quickly, making hypoglycaemia more likely. This means the leg should be avoided as an injection site for sports involving running and the arms avoided before a game of tennis.
- **Temperature**   High temperatures makes insulin work faster and low temperatures the opposite. This may be relevant with sports such as swimming outdoors or taking part in sports outdoors when it is hot.

Food

- **Extra carbohydrate**   This may be necessary before, during and/or after exercise to avoid hypoglycaemia, depending on the intensity and duration of the exercise. Discuss with your diabetes team the type of snacks needed, and whether your insulin regimen allows you to make adjustments to insulin doses to limit hypoglycaemia without taking extra food.

Exercise

- **Intensity** Light and moderate exercise lowers blood glucose usually within 20–60 minutes of the exercise and up to several hours later. Very strenuous exercise generally raises blood glucose because of the immediate release of the stress hormones adrenaline and cortisol. This effect normally lasts for 30–60 minutes but then the blood glucose will start to fall.
- **Duration** Exercising for more than 30 minutes will cause some kind of blood glucose drop unless there is not enough insulin on board.
- **Frequency** This is how often and regularly someone takes part in sport; muscles can stay more sensitive to the effects of the exercise for up to 2 days after sport. Regular exercise brings increased sensitivity to insulin generally, which may mean needing to adjust insulin doses less than irregular exercise. The opposite is true: if someone never does sport and then goes on an activity camp, blood glucose can drop dramatically. In this situation insulin doses will need to be reduced. The younger the child the more likely they are to exercise naturally every day, with fewer swings in blood glucose and less need for dose adjustments.
- **Timing** The body produces hormones, which increase blood glucose in the early morning so exercising then may cause blood glucose to rise, or make it less likely to fall.

Blood glucose

- **Blood glucose control** If control is poor, there may not be enough insulin on board and the 'counter-regulatory' hormone response, which occurs with exercise, will be more marked causing blood glucose to rise.
- **Blood glucose level** This may reflect the amount of insulin on board. It also affects how exertion is perceived.

Hypoglycaemia and exercise

When hypos occur the effect can last for up to 8 hours, sometimes even longer, because the muscles are still sensitive and glycogen stores in the liver and muscle, which normally break down to release glucose, are empty. This means that hypos may occur during and after sport, especially over night. So eating a larger snack before bed the night after exercise to refill those glycogen stores and keep up the blood sugars and/or reducing the evening insulin may be needed to avoid night-time hypos.

If hypoglycaemia is occurring with exercise it will be because the balance between the amounts of insulin, the level of activity and the carbohydrate intake is incorrect. This may be for one of the following reasons.

■ There is too much insulin around. If you are going to reduce insulin discuss this first with your diabetes team.

■ More than 30 minutes of moderate sport (or shorter if the exercise is more intense) usually causes blood glucose to start to fall. Taking an extra snack, such as a sports drink before and/or half-way through the sport may prevent this. If you have reduced insulin before exercise your child may not actually need an extra snack before sport, but may need it during the exercise and will need to stock up those glycogen stores after.

Hyperglycaemia

Sometimes, confusingly, blood glucose may rise with exercise in several situations:

■ Strenuous exercise, when blood glucose rises due to the release of stress hormones, glucagon and adrenaline;

■ If there is not enough insulin around, such as when an insulin injection has been missed or when exercise is taken before an evening injection is due if on a twice-a-day regimen;

■ Too large a snack is eaten for the amount of exercise;

■ In competitive sports where stress hormones are produced with the excitement of competition.

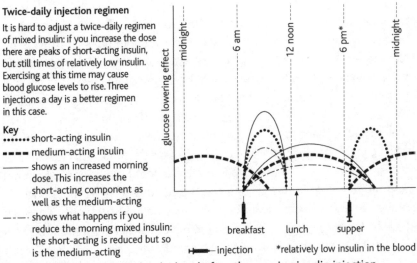

Twice-daily injection regimen

It is hard to adjust a twice-daily regimen of mixed insulin: if you increase the dose there are peaks of short-acting insulin, but still times of relatively low insulin. Exercising at this time may cause blood glucose levels to rise. Three injections a day is a better regimen in this case.

Key

•••••• short-acting insulin

▬ ▬ ▬ medium-acting insulin

───── shows an increased morning dose. This increases the short-acting component as well as the medium-acting

─ ·─ ·─ shows what happens if you reduce the morning mixed insulin: the short-acting is reduced but so is the medium-acting

⊢▬▬ injection   *relatively low insulin in the blood

Background insulin levels drop before the evening insulin injection

Case 1

Jason discusses blood testing

Introducing Jason, 27 years, diagnosed aged 7

The worst thing about clinics is being told off. You feel it's not your fault you have diabetes. You have to go to clinic to be told off for something you didn't want in the first place. Parents, teachers, doctors – they're all telling you off. It encourages you to be dishonest. Sometimes I would say 'everything's fine' just because I didn't want to discuss it. So if my HbA$_{1c}$ was high I didn't want to listen. It was a closed relationship.

Occasionally I made up test results. I was going to clinic and I hadn't done enough or I hadn't written them down. I made them vary with different handwriting styles and different coloured pens. I didn't mind doing the blood tests but sometimes I'd go long periods not doing any because I was thinking of other things. Then I'd get into the habit again.

As a child you think you can see the pattern. You think, 'What can they tell me that I don't already know?'

Discussion

Jason highlights some of the anxieties that young people with diabetes face: feeling that they are being criticised and constantly under scrutiny. Jason feels nagged by all those non-diabetic experts around him. He didn't actually mind doing the blood tests, it's just that he forgot sometimes. Jason felt that he could not be upfront about not having done enough blood tests to satisfy his doctors, or when he had, not having written them down. Instead he felt that he had to make them up. It's pretty easy for doctors and nurses to tell when patients do this as the blood test results in the book don't match their patient's HbA$_{1c}$. It's a shame that Jason felt he could not be open about not wanting to do blood tests at times, and forgetting to write them down at others, for fear of 'being told off'. If Jason could have been open he might have had a discussion about the problem and reached a solution. He may have just 'forgotten' when times were busy. Alternatively, it may have been a means of denial and shutting out reminders of his diabetes. Many of us with diabetes who feel ashamed about having high blood glucose results may not want to write the result down when they are 'bad' because then it is there in black and white: a reminder of the diabetes, the failure of having a high blood glucose level and all that it entails, which may be fear of complications or being told off or criticised.

Jason felt he had to lie and thereafter was not open to anything in the consultation. This seems a bit silly. After all, a blood glucose level is just the result of not giving enough insulin to match the amount of food intake in relation to activity levels. Starting to see blood glucose results in terms of cause and effect rather than as someone's fault would allow an open discussion.

Jason felt that the diabetes team couldn't add anything to his care and that he knew best. This is a common feeling amongst those of us with diabetes. In part this is true: after all, it is our body. When others offer up advice and dish out demands, it just reinforces our feeling that we are not understood. It is difficult to accept help when it involves more demanding care, especially if you don't feel unwell. However, it can be hard sometimes to see patterns and trends when you are immersed in it every day. Having someone to look at the whole picture can be helpful. The combination of an individual's unique perspective on their own diabetes (or as a parent, your child's diabetes) and a doctor's general experience of managing many people's diabetes, has the potential to be a strong partnership.

Getting into a regular routine from the start with blood testing is important. It should become part of the normal daily routine. After all, you wouldn't leave the house without putting on your underwear or brushing your teeth; or would you?

Wake up
   Wash hands
      Blood test
         Shower
            Get dressed
               Injection
                  Breakfast
                     Brush teeth
                        Catch the bus to school

The morning rush

Q Joe gets upset when his blood sugar is high. We do too. I try to follow all the advice but we still seem to get it wrong. When can I expect things to get easier?

A It can feel like a constant battle to try and get your child's blood glucose level in the correct range. Even if you follow all the advice, you will still find that the blood test result is unpredictable and the diabetes is always one step ahead of you. Sometimes it can feel as if there is no rhyme or reason to the blood glucose level at all.

Blood glucose is regulated and affected by so many different things that it can be difficult to tease out the reasons for a blood glucose result, but there will always be one. Trying to take all the variables affecting blood glucose into account at one time seems nearly impossible when you think about it. So when you do manage it, it can seem like a real achievement.

For those of you reading this who do not have diabetes, your body will be making intricate changes all the time to keep your blood glucose level in the normal range. In those of us who do have diabetes, the only regulators of blood glucose that can be controlled are insulin, food and exercise. Having said all that, with time and personal experience you and your child will become expert at looking back and finding an explanation for the blood glucose result. This is what will help you in the future to make adjustments, by planning the amount of insulin needed depending on your child's activity level, food intake and current health, rather than reacting to the result. In other words it is important to anticipate ahead of time what will be required, being 'proactive' rather than 'reactive'. As you and your child get better at being proactive, you will become the experts of your child's diabetes. It may seem a long way away now but it is only just around the corner when you will feel expert in making the decisions.

Learning to be proactive rather than purely reactive involves thinking about when you have done the blood test. Don't forget that the blood glucose level that you check is just a snapshot of a single moment in time. If you have done it straight after a meal

A *continued*

the blood glucose level is going to be high. However, it shouldn't be too high 1½–2 hours after eating, so if you want to check your child's blood glucose level after eating, it is best to wait until 1½–2 hours have passed or you might correct it unnecessarily and bring on a hypo.

There is always a risk that focusing in too much detail on the blood glucose results may make you and your child start worrying when it is out of range. If you then act on a high result by restricting food or doing an injection it can feel like a punishment. Some children get really upset about high blood glucose levels and can feel like they are 'bad diabetics'. They will have been told what number is 'good' and what number is 'bad', and you will have been told, too. Your child may become upset at disappointing you and their doctors as well as themselves. They may feel it is easier just to avoid doing them or not write the high ones down in the record book. Of course it is important to try and get the blood glucose level as near normal as possible without too many hypos, but ideally also without obsessing too much about them. A healthy interest and willingness to want to think about and act on the results is all that is needed, otherwise your child may just start to feel like they are a number. You will never be able to get the blood glucose level 'perfect' all of the time and if you expect this, or doctors expect this of their patients, everyone will be frustrated and unhappy.

I remember one diabetic camp where I was the doctor looking after a large group of children aged 7–11. We were all doing our blood test before the evening meal and the children were coming up to talk to me so we could decide together how much insulin they needed. One girl walked up slowly and stood next to me holding her blood test book in both hands. Her eyes were brimming with tears and she was looking at her shoes. I asked her what was wrong. 'I'm 27 and I don't know why', she said. She was devastated and felt a complete failure at having such a high blood glucose result. After some hugs and tissues she still ate her supper and joined in the evening activity. She has always stuck in my mind as I talk with children and parents about doing blood tests.

Whatever I do, I never seem to get it right.
(Chantelle, 12)

My mum gets all stressy and is like 'WHY are they high?' Sometimes your sugars like to piss you off. You've been really 'good' and you check your sugars and bam, they're '17mmols', and while you're annoyed about that yourself, the last thing you need is someone just as stressy and asking WHY?
(Juliet, 22)

If my blood's between 5 and 7 [mmol/l] it's my sense of achievement in life. I feel immense satisfaction. It makes you feel like you've done something right.
(Ruth, 38)

My first doctor told me it was bad to eat certain things and bad to have a high blood sugar. If I had a high blood test I felt guilty, I thought it was something I had done. No one in my family gave me a hard time about eating certain foods but I was quite hard on myself and gave myself a bit of a guilt trip. I've only just broken the cycle.
(Flin, 23)

Q I'm trying to encourage Bev to take more responsibility by doing blood tests herself. She will do some but not all of them and never writes them down. How can I get her to be more involved?

A Blood tests make up the bulk of the monotony of having diabetes. Some children genuinely forget about doing blood tests as they have other things going on. It can also seem like 'a hassle'. It's easy to get fed up, especially if there doesn't seem to be any good reason for their blood glucose result. Also, if the blood glucose level is just a bit high then your child will probably feel completely healthy and

continued

therefore will have no motivation to try and bring the level down. When you think about it, if your child doesn't like knowing their blood glucose level is out of range then the easiest thing to avoid the hyperglycaemia is not to do a test, or if you do it, not to write it down. By not doing a blood test, it is a guarantee that your child as well as you and your diabetes team will not know that they've had a high glucose level. This denial can be seen in other aspects of diabetes care, from missing injections to eating unhealthily.

Children will have more pressing things on their minds to think about. However, as they get older and become more aware of their bodies, the hope is that they will become interested in their blood glucose levels too. For young children, who will rely on you to do most of their tests, the transition to when they are fully self-testing can be gradual. Even young children can take part in some of the blood test, such as throwing the used strips away or turning on the machine.

It can bemuse medical teams why those with diabetes test their blood but don't write down the results. It's easier to understand when you think how much time it takes up cumulatively. However, in the long run it can be almost impossible to see a trend and then make appropriate changes without the written record. One way around this is to get a blood testing machine that can be linked to a computer which can then download the readings and print them to show the trends.

Many school-age children, as well as adults, think they can predict their blood glucose level without doing a blood test. However, these predictions can be misleading. Tiredness can be misinterpreted as being high or low. Also, someone who normally runs their blood glucose level in the higher range may feel hypo when their blood glucose is normal or even a bit high. It is possible for those with diabetes to feel 'absolutely normal' with blood glucose levels that are a bit on the high side. If this goes on for a long time, there will be the risk of complications. Also, many people who then decide to be more interested in their blood glucose levels or have a reason for tighter control, such as preparing for a sporting event or getting

continued on next page

A *continued*

pregnant, will say that although they didn't think they felt unwell before, now that their blood glucose levels are lower they feel so much better, in terms of energy levels and general well-being.

The only way to get children doing their own blood tests is to make them interested in knowing what the result will be, by understanding that what they do will influence the result of the blood glucose level and how they feel. Then the light bulb goes on and there is a reason for doing the boringly annoying blood test and it becomes something of interest and of importance. However, this can be difficult to maintain when other things come up in life. Sometimes you will all just need a day off. Try to help children like Bev by remaining positive; encourage and praise good behaviour, and just ignore bad behaviour. This will go a long way to helping children feel encouraged and stop them feeling they are being criticised and that they are a failure.

I feel funny then I do a test.

(Chantelle, 12)

If I'm high or low I don't bother doing it because I know I'm low or high. I forget to do it, especially at school. Sometimes I get annoyed...it can take five times before I get enough blood.

(Janina, 13)

I feel so lousy if I'm high. Sometimes you just can't tell unless you do a test. I was on a trip. I was thirsty and feeling nauseous. I was all set to do an injection but my blood was 6.8 [mmol/l].

(Lucia, 37)

Initially I thought blood testing was only something that happened in hospital. I do them every so often if I feel hypo or high. I just can't be bothered. I don't have much foresight. I look to tomorrow, not to the future. I'd like to get good end results without having to do the test. I think I can judge in my head what my blood sugar is.

(Luke, 17)

I can't tell if I'm high or low so I have to check.

(David, 11)

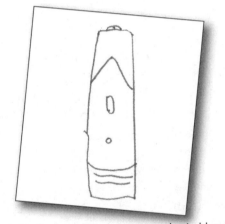

A child drew the fingerpricker she uses to obtain blood for testing at home.

Q The diabetes team want Freddie to test his blood up to four times a day but it hurts him and it's so stressful to get him to do it. Do I have to?

A Anyone who has a fingerprick blood test will feel the needle, or 'pricker', going into their finger. However, if done correctly using the sides rather than the fleshy bit of the finger and the minimum depth of the needle, it causes only a small bit of discomfort. In days gone by the needles were quite thick and there was no depth adjustment on the fingerpricking device and still people agreed to test their blood glucose levels at home.

continued on next page

A *continued*

Don't use the same site for fingerpricking again and again. Use one finger one day, and a different finger the next: in other words, rotate the sites. This is important because otherwise thick skin will build up and the fingers may get sore. Many children test their blood using the same fingers and they develop thick skin which then doesn't hurt. However it is unsightly to see finger calluses and it can reduce finger sensation. This is why you shouldn't use the thumb and first fingers on the dominant hand (the right hand if right-handed or the left if left-handed), which we rely on to pick things up. You could also try using earlobes as a break.

If it hurts your child to do a blood test speak to your diabetes specialist nurse and check you are using the finest needle that is available. There are also different types of fingerpricking devices that can be used with various different prickers. Some are better than others and given the choice, your child will have their favourite, or best, their least unfavourite. There are also prickers that can use other bits of the skin like the forearms.

I suggest you give Freddie the choice from a range of devices available. It will allow him a sense of taking control of his diabetes, rather than having diabetes imposed upon him. You should also remind yourself what it feels like. Maybe you can try them out together (but you should not share the same fingerpricking device). At the end of the day you and your child will need to find something that suits you both because if you don't test the blood glucose level, you will not know what it is. Knowing what your child's blood glucose level is will be important if you are to make adjustments for variations in appetite and activity levels. This will enable your child to be full of energy and less likely to develop complications in the long term.

If you make a big deal about the blood tests, so will your child. Listen to what your child says – if it hurts, believe him, check for yourself and see what else is available. No one likes being told what they 'have' to do, especially if it hurts. Your child will feel much happier when the decisions come from him. Be careful though – you also don't want to let yourself be manipulated. All children want to see how far they can push the boundaries with parents. Try not to start

continued

bribing them into doing their blood test or you could be penniless this time next year! However, flattery, a reward system and positive encouragement will take you a long way.

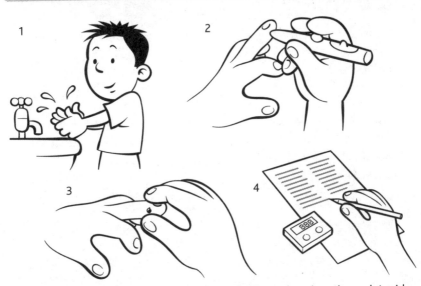

Take blood for testing from the sides of the fingers rather than the pad. Avoid the thumb and first finger of the dominant hand.

In the first two years I was strict. After that I used to make up my blood tests, I couldn't be arsed to test. I used to say I had sore fingers as an excuse.

(George, 35)

I have a phobia of blood. I fret to do even one blood test a year. At the beginning it was a big deal even to do a fingerprick. My tolerance grew: it was something I had to do.

(Daniel, 17)

I worry about my fingers – there's so little space there. It's a means to an end – there's no other way of measuring it [the blood glucose]. It hurts my fingers and is more painful than injections.

(Beatrice, 31)

I test my forearm and it doesn't hurt at all.

(Summer, 13)

I used to hate doing blood tests when I was younger, it hurt and it was an inconvenience. I didn't rotate my sites. Now I've lost sensation in the sides of my fingers. It's still a pain but it's always a great excuse to have nice big handbags.

(Katherine, 30)

At the beginning I did my blood tests a lot. My fingers used to get so rough it was hard to get blood out of me.

(Daniel, 17)

I used to do the tips of my fingers which was a problem as I played the piano and violin. Then I was told to do the sides of my fingers and it's been fine. It hasn't affected my sensitivity at all.

(Mike, 27)

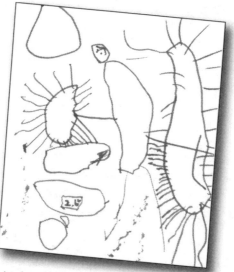

Patrick, 4, drew his hands. The 'pins' are actually his fingers. His mother says that they call his fingerpricks 'having his finger done' so maybe Patrick thinks he has rather a lot of fingers done.

Q **Fiona checks her blood about six times a day but her HbA$_{1c}$ is still high. It doesn't seem to be helping. How come we still manage to get it wrong?**

A Many people with diabetes can get into the habit of 'just checking' blood glucose levels. It can be a relief to know what the level is. It's easy to get a bit obsessional about doing blood tests, especially if you are worried about having hypos. Your child might be relieved to be running a bit high just to avoid them.

If Fiona is checking her blood a lot and her HbA$_{1c}$ is still high, I wonder if she is writing the results down. If she is, then is anyone acting on what they see? If the blood result isn't being written down it seems a shame when most of the hard work has already been done. Perhaps you could take some of the effort from Fiona by writing down the blood test result at the end of the day using the machine's memory function, or downloading her blood test machine onto the computer. If you, together with your diabetes team, look at the results you may be able to see a trend and make some changes for the better. Then when the blood glucose levels improve you and Fiona will see and feel the benefits.

I wish I could just look at a machine and know what my blood was. Sometimes I just go into a panic and I can't even get my blood test out to check in case I'm hypo.

(Jane, 34)

I test my blood three to five times a day. I don't always pay it the attention from a wider angle that it warrants but I always correct my blood sugar when it's high.

(Beatrice, 31)

What you can do

- **Make sure you have a fingerpricking device** in which you can adjust the depth of the needle, and the finest fingerpricking needle that works in the device. Ask your diabetes specialist nurse regularly as new products are always becoming available.

- **Check your technique.** Make sure you know how to do the blood test as painlessly and accurately as possible. This means making sure fingers are not covered with anything that might artificially give you high glucose reading, such as fruit or Frosties, and that any washed fingers are dry, as damp fingers can give you an artificially low reading. Remember to use the sides of the fingers and avoid the thumb and first finger.

- **Practise on yourself** before you practise on your child. If your child is young they can practise on dolls or teddies. Show them that you are not scared by letting them fingerprick you too.

- **Find out about blood testing machines.** To my knowledge, there are machines that take 3 seconds to read a blood test, can store up to 30 days' worth of blood glucose levels, can be downloaded onto a computer and work out averages. When I was diagnosed 23 years ago, it took 3 minutes to check your blood glucose on a machine the size of a small shoe. Now I can take my blood testing machine and a couple of test strips in my pocket when I go for a jog. I look forward to giving in the next edition a description of an even smaller, faster and sexier piece of kit.

- **Avoid blame.** Finding a reason to blame someone for a 'good' or 'bad' blood glucose test result, whether it is you, your partner, your child or someone else, will be soul-destroying. Instead try to think of the blood glucose result in terms of cause and effect in order to learn from it for next time.

- **Make adjustments for sport**. Getting blood glucose levels right is important to avoid hypos as well as hypers. You should discuss with your diabetes team the type of sport your child wants to take part in. Reducing insulin doses too much or taking too large a snack to avoid hypos can mean high blood glucose levels, which worsen blood glucose control and impair performance and enjoyment with sport.

There are a few simple rules.
- Think about and discuss the issues with your diabetes team.
- Do a blood test before sport; if it is over 14 mmol/l and the last insulin injection was several hours ago it may mean that there is not enough insulin around and the blood glucose may rise with exercise. Check ketones, and if positive sport may need to be delayed and some insulin given, especially if there is thirst, feeing sick or tummy ache, all of which are signs of ketones being present.
- Discuss with your diabetes team whether you should be changing insulin doses or if a snack is needed before or during sport.
- Have a larger bedtime snack after exercising and watch out for hypos the next day too.
- Make sure you test before bed after sport. I usually recommend keeping the blood glucose above 7 mmol/l before bed, especially after exercise.
- Teenagers should avoid alcohol or take an even larger snack after exercising because alcohol stops new glucose being produced and so hypos are more likely, especially overnight.
- For those interested in competitive or endurance training, further information can found from the website **Runsweet** (www. runsweet.com). There are some centres being set up in the UK that specialise in this area so ask your diabetes team about it, as you may be able to be referred. Diabetes does not need to prevent your child becoming a 2012 or 2016 Olympic medal winner.

Rachel's view

'I'm more than just a number.'

I feel upset and annoyed when I hear children talking about the guilt they feel when their blood glucose is high. Who makes them feel like that? It's not their fault they have diabetes, and assigning blame doesn't help. What does help, however, is understanding where the level came from and providing motivation to improve it. I know this from personal experience as I used to – and still do – get wrapped up in the 'numbers game'. I care what my blood glucose is now and for my future and get cross with myself when I don't get it right. It is hard work at times and requires thought which is time-consuming and tiring. But it also reaps benefits to me since I feel better and can do more, and then have to put less time into my diabetes. Thinking about blood glucose results in terms of cause and effect, rather than guilt and blame, has really helped me to objectively analyse my blood test results from a more distant viewpoint. The opportunity also to re-educate myself, through writing this book, has resulted in my HbA_{1c} dropping by a whole percentage point and my blood glucose levels have become a lot more predictable.

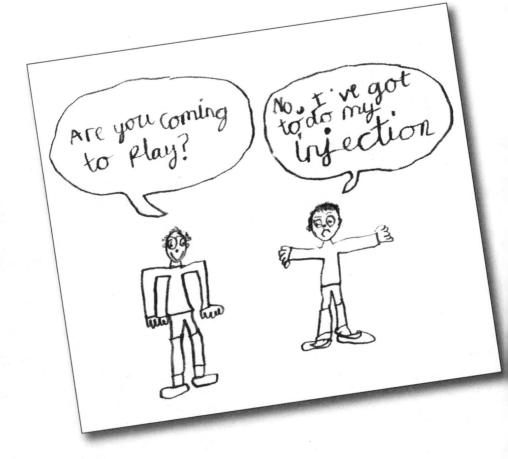

4

Injection time

What is insulin?

Insulin is a hormone, one of the body's many chemical messengers. Hormones are produced by endocrine glands and go around the body in the bloodstream. The pancreas, which lies behind the stomach, has glandular tissue that makes and releases insulin. The pancreas cells that produce insulin are the beta cells which are grouped in clusters called the islets of Langerhans (after the doctor who identified them). The islets also contain alpha cells which produce glucagon, one of the important hormones that can raise blood glucose (see Chapter 2).

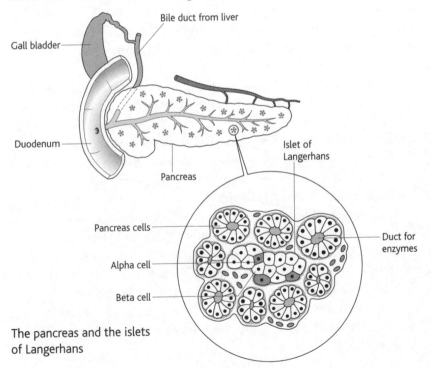

The pancreas and the islets of Langerhans

How does insulin work and what does it do?

Insulin acts in several different ways with the overall effect of lowering the level of glucose in the blood. It keeps the body's energy stores in balance, by allowing glucose to enter the body's cells where it can be used for energy. Without insulin the body's muscle and fat stores start to break down to release energy causing ketones to be produced which make the blood more acidic than it should be.

What insulins are available to people with diabetes?

There are many different types of insulin that vary in their speed of action and how long they last in the body.

Regular, short-acting insulin is the type of insulin that is closest to natural insulin. It is also called **soluble insulin**. Analogue insulins are a variety of newer insulins in which the structure of insulin has been altered to change its properties, such as how quickly it starts to work and how long its effects last. Regular, short-acting insulin takes 30 minutes to 1 hour to start working, peaks in 2–4 hours and lasts 5–8 hours, e.g. actrapid. This insulin is most often used when intravenous insulin is needed in hospital at diagnosis, or if your child is unwell and producing ketones.

Rapid-acting analogue insulins start sooner and peak earlier than regular insulin but do not last as long (up to 3–5 hours), e.g. aspart (NovoRapid®), glulisine (Apidra®), lispro (Humalog®). Since they work quickly they can be given just before, during or after eating. They are useful to correct a sudden high blood glucose level, or when your child wants a sweet treat. These insulins are also used in insulin pumps. Except for insulin pumps, they must be used in conjunction with longer-acting insulins.

Medium-acting insulins are used as part of a once-daily or twice-daily regimen, e.g. isophane insulin (Humulin I®) and Insulatard.

Long-acting analogue insulins last up to 24 hours and are given once or twice a day, e.g. detemir (Levemir®), glargine (Lantus®). They can be used with rapid-acting insulins which are given at mealtimes.

Mixed insulins combine short-acting and long-acting insulins, e.g. aspart (NovoMix® 30) has 30% short-acting and the rest is medium- to long-acting insulin.

Name	Manufacturer	Taken
Rapid-acting insulins		
NovoRapid	Novo Nordisk	*Just before, with or just after food*
Humalog	Lilly	*Just before, with or just after food*
Medium-acting insulins		
Insulatard	Novo Nordisk	*About 30 minutes before food or bed*
Humulin I	Lilly	*About 30 minutes before food or bed*
Long-acting insulins		
Lantus	Sanofi-Aventis	*Once a day, any time (but the same time each day)*
Levemir	Novo Nordisk	*Once or twice daily*
Mixed insulins		
Mixtard 30	Novo Nordisk	*30 minutes before food*
Humalog Mix 25	Lilly	*Just before/with/just after food*
Humalog Mix 50	Lilly	*Just before/with/just after food*
NovoMix 30	Novo Nordisk	*Just before/with/just after food*
Short-acting insulin		
Actrapid	Novo Nordisk	*30 minutes before food*

The types of insulin most commonly used in children

Where can insulin be injected?

Insulin needs to be injected into fatty tissue, so any area that has fat under the skin can be injected. However, the depth of the fat as well as the type of insulin will affect how fast the insulin is soaked up into the blood (absorbed). The usual injection sites are:

■ the tummy;

■ the front and side of the thigh;

■ the upper outer part of the buttock; and

■ the sides of the upper arm.

These are good sites as they avoid hitting nerves and blood vessels. To remember the best place to inject in the buttock, imagine a cross dividing each buttock into four quarters, and use to upper outer quarter.

The different sites are useful in different situations. For example, the tummy has a more predictable absorption and is useful when faster insulin absorption is needed; the thighs and bottom are useful for the

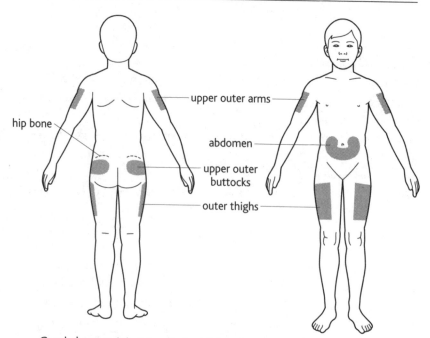

Good places to inject insulin in children. In young and particularly lean children, you may need to avoid the arms and tummy as there may not be enough fat there.

long-acting injections since insulin is absorbed more slowly from these sites. The arms can only be used in a child who has enough fat to avoid injecting into a muscle.

It is important to get insulin injection technique correct to reduce pain and make sure insulin is delivered properly. If insulin is injected into a muscle it may be painful, cause bruising and also lead to insulin being absorbed into the body too quickly and acting too quickly.

It is also important to rotate injection sites. Injecting the same sites causes fat to be broken down (lipoatrophy) or built up (lipohypertrophy). This looks unsightly and also leads to insulin being used unreliably, causing erratic blood glucose levels.

What are the different ways insulin can be given?

The standard way of giving insulin is by injection through the skin into the fat underneath, or if in hospital, through a drip into a vein. Inhaled insulin is no longer available in the UK at the time of writing this book. It was previously only licensed for adults.

1 Twice-daily injections

Usually with 'mixed insulin', which comprises a short-acting insulin and a medium-acting insulin, which lasts longer.

This regimen suits younger children and those with a predictable routine. It can be too restrictive for children who need flexibility, such as in size of meals, and those doing sports.

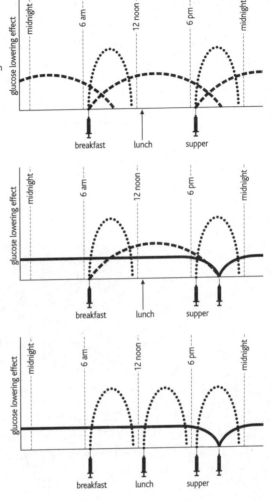

2 Three injections a day

Mixed insulin at breakfast, some short-acting insulin at dinnertime and a long-acting insulin once a day, either morning or evening.

This regimen is popular with school age children as it avoids a lunchtime injection.

3 Four injections a day ('basal bolus' regimen)

A long-acting insulin once a day ('basal') plus short-acting insulin with meals/large snacks ('bolus'). Although there are more injections, this is a flexible regimen, especially in timing of meals.

A basal bolus regimen of 4 or 5 injections a day suits carbohydrate counting (see p. 97), as do insulin pumps.

4 Five injections a day

Morning and evening injections of long-acting insulin, plus short-acting insulin at mealtimes and for large snacks.

This regimen is for those who find a long-acting insulin once a day does not last a full 24 hours.

Key

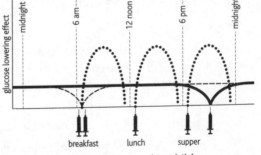

—— long-acting insulin
- - - - 2nd long-acting insulin
■■■■ medium-acting insulin
•••••• short-acting insulin
┣━━ injection

These are the regimens of injecting insulin mostly used in children.

There most common methods of injecting insulin are:

■ a disposable plastic syringe;
■ a 'pen' device containing a prefilled insulin cartridge; or
■ an insulin pump.

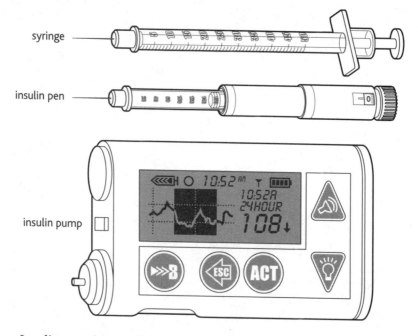

Insulin pens have a dial on which you can set the correct dose. There are audible clicks in some pens. Some pens have automatic injector devices and a cover which hides the needle so it can't be seen when entering the skin.

Other ways of taking insulin through the skin

Jet injector

There is a jet injector which can deliver insulin through the skin without a needle, powered through the skin using a jet of air. However, some people find this as painful as injections, or even more painful, and it can cause bruising; but it can be useful for those with a severe needle phobia. It is also possible to use a device which lies under the skin called a subcutaneous indwelling catheter, e.g. Insuflon. This is inserted using a needle into the fat layer below the skin and then the needle is removed leaving a short plastic tube, like a small straw, through which insulin can be given. It needs to be changed every couple of days.

Insulin pump

An insulin pump also delivers insulin into the fat under the skin. A short fat syringe which holds enough fast-acting insulin for 2–3 days sits in a small box that can be clipped onto a belt. This is connected through a piece of plastic tubing into the fat layer under the skin, again introduced through a small needle that is then removed. A small amount of rapid-acting insulin is delivered continuously, with more insulin being released when the user sets it to do so, such as after eating carbohydrate-containing food. The needle site needs to be changed every 2–3 days or fatty lumps can start to build up.

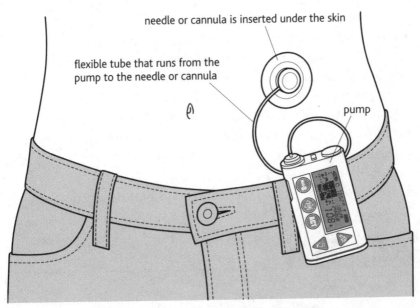

needle or cannula is inserted under the skin

flexible tube that runs from the pump to the needle or cannula

pump

This is how an insulin pump looks when worn.

It is easy to change the rates of insulin delivery to suit different times of the day. For example, a child may need a different rate of insulin at night than during the day. Different rates may also be needed for shorter periods of time, for example if blood glucose readings are running a bit high during an illness or menstruation; the rate may also be reduced before, during or after sport.

With a pump, you need to count the amount of carbohydrate you eat (or your child eats) and give a certain amount of insulin to match. The insulin can also be given in different ways depending on the type of carbohydrate. For example, you can choose to give the insulin over several hours for a slow-releasing carbohydrate such as pasta, or straight away if eating a piece of fruit.

What affects how quickly insulin works?

The speed of action varies a great deal between individuals, and even in the same person on different days.

These are the factors that affect how quickly insulin works.

■ Insulin: faster-acting insulins are absorbed faster.
■ Fat layer: the thinner the child, the thinner the fat layer and the faster the insulin works.
■ Age: younger children have less fat and so the insulin works faster.
■ Injection site: insulin works faster when injected incorrectly into muscle rather than fat; injecting into the tummy is faster than the thigh, except with glargine.
■ Lipohypertrophy: the build-up of fat slows down insulin absorption.
■ Insulin dose: the smaller the amount of insulin, the faster it is absorbed.
■ Exercise: this increases insulin activity, particularly when injecting in the working muscle.
■ Temperature: higher temperatures both outside and in the body increase insulin absorption.

Case 1

First injection

Introducing Lizzie, 27, diagnosed aged 8

I was led into a side room with polished pale blue tiles. You could make out the reflection of the grey plastic couch and the window, held slightly ajar. On one side of the room was a shelf with boxes of different sizes, underneath which were mauve cupboards and a small white fridge. The walls were white interrupted by a picture painted by someone called Alice. 'I love Marion' was written over the top of

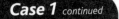

Case 1 *continued*

the picture of a stick-girl painted in yellow and pink. I sat on the couch for a few seconds whilst Marion left the room and returned with an orange and syringe. She had done my injection yesterday and this morning, whilst I had practised on an orange. This time it was my turn.

Mum silently kept guard on the inside of the door making sure no one could enter. Marion pinched up the skin on my thigh a bit and I pulled off the syringe lid. I remember seeing the needle glisten in the light and wondering how I could push it through my skin. I held it really close so it made a dent in the skin on my thigh and then pulled away. Marion and I counted to three together and with her hand over mine the needle slid in. My hand was shaking so it was difficult to hold the needle with one hand and reach for the plunger with the other. Marion held the syringe for me and I pushed in the clear liquid. The needle came out and I rubbed my leg. I looked down and saw that where the needle had been was now a tiny empty hole filling with a pool of clear liquid. I smiled and looked at Mum who smiled with tears in her eyes and told me she was proud of me.

Discussion

Many people who do not understand diabetes associate it solely with injections. You will know that there is more to it than that. Injections – how often, where, how much and (for some) how to adjust the dose – are certainly a part of your child's everyday life. On top of that come balancing food, exercise, hypos, hypers, school, family life and normal childhood illnesses.

Injections are crucial; they are the only reliable way of giving the body what is missing, insulin. So issues surrounding injections are important.

The first injection is often a landmark occasion for you and your child. Lizzie in Case 1 can clearly remember her first injection 19 years on, despite having administered 20,000 or so injections so far in her lifetime. Many children adapt easily to injections and soon get used to them. Others, however, especially younger children, fear injections and find them painful. Having said that, people often overreact to having inject-ions. They really are pretty easy with the sharp needles used today – most injections you don't actually feel at all. As children get older, their fears and sensitivities around their diabetes change, although a few teenagers still find the pain close to unbearable.

The average age for learning to self-inject is around nine years of age, although the variation is very wide. Even when a child can do their own injection, you may need to take back the responsibility when it becomes too much, until your child feels able to take it on again. Of course you will want your child to do their own injections, but doing your child's injection yourself, although it may sound strange, is part of an intimate physical bond between you and your child: like washing and dressing them. Once this is removed you may feel like they have 'grown up' to some degree, and just like any growing-up process, this can be emotionally challenging for a parent.

Lizzie seemed to be ready to inject herself from the beginning. Whilst this should be encouraged, it can be harmful to push a child who is not ready. Children expect and need their parents to look after them. With age, they take on new responsibilities for themselves. Injecting is one such responsibility and there is no 'right time' for this.

Case 2

Finding places to do injections

Introducing Kiet, 16, diagnosed aged 15

On the streets there's nowhere for you to do your injection. People will think you're a drug addict.

I was in a chip shop with my friends, sitting down doing my injection. The man in the shop said, 'If you're going to do that don't do it in here'. He started shouting and called the manager. Now I eat if I'm out and do my injection at home. If I'm in a restaurant I go to the toilet to do it. People stare and laugh at me.

I don't mind doing the injection, it's just the point of doing it before you eat. When you're really hungry you want to eat straight away, you don't want to wait and do your injection.

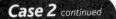

Case 2 *continued*

At school I had to leave lessons early and go to the Medical Room to do my blood test and injection. I was told to inject and eat in there. I had to do it for two weeks. I got bored of it. I said, 'It's my life and you can't do nothing about it'. I'd rather do it without anyone knowing. I can't do it in school, as the toilets are broken. I don't inject in school any more so my bloods are high.

Discussion

For the older child who demands a greater flexibility in their life, like Kiet, the trouble caused by injecting before you eat or injecting in a public place is worse than the actual injection.

Kiet has had some bad experiences injecting in public. Injecting in a lavatory does not seem a hygienic practice and is often not advised by healthcare professionals. If you ask children and adults with diabetes, I expect most will say they have injected in lavatories in the past. Many still do when they are out in a public place, or in the company of people without diabetes, and have no problems whatsoever. This might horrify you, but bear in mind that injecting in public may bring unwanted attention and it can be less trouble in the long run just to sneak away to the toilets. Whilst privacy is important, injecting in public should also not be a reason to be ashamed. If it means that your child has to take time away from other activities, such as missing lesson time in school or being late for lunch, this needs to be addressed. The important thing is how the young person with diabetes feels about it: whether they are happy to inject in public or want to inject somewhere private like the toilets.

One way of making injecting less noticeable is to use different sites for the injections. For example, injecting in the tummy is practical at the meal table and at school.

Since Kiet's blood glucose may not be raised before eating and he feels well, he may not understand the importance of injecting close to his meal. A delayed injection may soon become a missed one, leading to hyperglycaemia which brings its own difficulties (see Chapter 6).

Case 3

A mother compares injections then and now

Five years ago when my daughter was four we were using syringes and drawing up insulin. I was so traumatised with it all. It seemed surreal, standing in the kitchen practising injecting an orange with a syringe. I remember shaking with fear trying not to get the air bubbles in this horrendous needle I associated with drug addicts. I cried for months. Thankfully, after a few months the pen came along. I was so relieved. It radically changed me and the way I was dealing with the condition.

Last September my daughter took the initiative to start injecting herself. She now has so many more options for trips, sleepovers, teas and countless other activities. However, it has been a long road emotionally. I tried early last year and she was very afraid and tearful. I was conscious it wasn't the right time but laid the foundations for later. I think meeting other children and making a diabetic friend who was already injecting herself meant that she talked it over with her. She started to say that she might try, but it took a year. Now she is doing a better job than me with no bleeding or bruising. Sometimes she refuses to do her injection. I leave her for a while and we negotiate and she eats first and then injects.

As we have gone on we have developed our own routine. Injections happen, teeth-brushing happens and getting ready for school happens. It's so much part of our life it is hard to believe we went through those painful early traumatic days. Often I say to her, 'When you are doing your injections, Mummy is taking out her contact lenses', something which I find a bore.

Discussion

The mother in Case 3 acknowledges that she has feelings about her child's diabetes. When the pen came along it made her life easier, perhaps a reflection of also making her child's life easier. She describes going through the process of trying to encourage her daughter to self-inject, having slowly to introduce the idea, back off and wait until she was ready.

It is important that you do not push a child to self-inject when they are not ready for that responsibility. Diabetes can skew development, making children act older than their years by taking on responsibilities that are more adult in nature.

For you, injections may bring a lack of spontaneity. Everything may seem like a big issue, especially at the beginning. Rest assured, it will get easier.

I remember the first time that my son bled after I had injected him, I sobbed and sobbed.

(A mother)

Q **Sam is eight and can do his own injections but sometimes he misses them and says that he has done it already. Why does he miss them when he ends up feeling ill?**

A Often young children hate the physical aspect of having injections – after all it is a needle going through their skin with nerve endings under the surface. Older children often 'get used' to the injections. Perhaps that is because the skin has toughened up, or because the needle is no longer being aimed at a moving target, or because the fear of a needle breaking their skin has subsided.

Many of the newer insulins can be injected just before, during or straight after eating, and the dose can be adjusted according to how much your child eats. Examples of these are aspart (NovoRapid®) and lispro (Humalog®). However, Sam may not be on these newer insulins since they involve four injections a day. Also, he might have been told to inject just before eating to avoid raised blood glucose levels after the meal.

Injecting before eating can be a hassle: it interrupts what you are doing. You just want to be eating and others are already tucking in. Many people with diabetes do not like injecting in front of other people because of the questions that are asked and the looks you get. At school, having to find somewhere to inject discreetly out of others' sight can mean you end up at the back of the dinner queue. If, like Kiet in Case 2, there isn't anywhere to do it, it might be

continued on next page

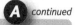

A *continued*

delayed or skipped completely. Others may opt for injecting through clothing which can be unreliable depending on where the needle reaches.

If you are hungry, the last thing you want is to have to do a blood test and inject. However, this needs to become routine and 'normal', even though it isn't part of other people's daily routine. If this is how Sam feels, there are ways around it, such as seeing if it is possible to change insulins so he can inject after eating. However, if this is not the reason for skipping the injection, it may be that Sam is trying to reject the fact that he has diabetes.

A point to remember is that when it comes to injection time a child will not be feeling unwell and will not feel like 'a diabetic'. But if they do skip the injection and become hyperglycaemic, then they may feel unwell and feel like they do have an illness. Perhaps Sam is getting fed up with the injections and wants some time off. It might be time for you to take over his injections for a while to give him a break.

Sometimes when I put my injection in it really hurts and I bleed.

(Margaret, 12)

I'd rather inject through my clothes than make a big deal about it. I don't like people gawping; it's too much.

(George, 35)

I hate it when people say 'You must be used to your injections by now'. Just because I prick myself four times a day doesn't mean I get used to it. You do get used to having to do it, but not to doing it. It's a bit like brushing your teeth.

(Beatrice, 31)

People start screaming if they see me do my injection. Then I get into trouble.

(Tom, 11)

Q Debbie is nine and only lets me do her injections. She is reluctant to try for herself. I have told her that it will stop her going to sleepovers but nothing will get her to try. How can I make her more independent?

A It can be a big step when children do their own injection for the first time, not only for them but also for you as a parent. Finally your child is moving on and growing up. All children like attention from their parents, and quality time together. Injection time can be a special 'you and me' time. They will be gaining independence by self-injecting but they will also be gaining new responsibilities, and with that comes a loss of freedom. It also may hit them that now it is up to them to do it for ever.

Some children may find it easier to start by sharing the responsibility. The first step is taking part in the injection process, even just taking off the pen lid. Slowly they may progress to dialling up the insulin and holding the pen with you. From here, they may move on to doing their injection for the first time. Sometimes, knowing that a parent is willing to take back the responsibility from them when they need a break, is what they need to help them take that step. Later, when they are doing the injections for themselves regularly, they may still feel totally fed up with endlessly having to do injections. Being able to take back the responsibility from them and give it back when the time is right may be just what your child needs in order to overcome the barriers and confront the realisation that they need to take on their diabetes long-term when the time comes.

It may be technically more difficult, particularly if your child is very young, to hold the skin with one hand and inject with the other. Practice makes perfect.

Pushing children to self-inject when they are not ready is never right. However, some young people might be ready to inject for themselves before you realise it and need a bit of a push. That incentive may be by seeing other children their age injecting themselves, in clinic or at a diabetes club or holiday.

Most of the time I don't feel it. Sometimes it hurts and leaves bruises. I remember when I was little it took me ages to do an injection. I was so scared. It hurts less when Mum does it. I will do my leg when I'm older and Mum refuses to do it. I won't want to show my bum any more.

(Janina, 13 years)

One friend fainted when he saw me doing my injection.

(Darren, 12)

I was a bit shocked when I moved from two to three, and then three to four injections a day. I started doing my injections and then I stopped because I got fed up. When you grow up you don't want your parents doing your injection. Now I use my legs of a night-time, belly the rest of the time. Mum used to do my bottom and arms but they got lumpy.

(Margaret, 12)

I've never let anyone do my injection for me since I was diagnosed. I know how to do it and can stop if it hurts and try again.

(Lizzie, 27)

Q My son is four and was diagnosed when he was two. He is too young to understand why I hold and jab him with a needle. How can I stop him thinking I am punishing him?

A This sounds very distressing for you, but it may not be so distressing for your son. Most children do not blame their parents for their diabetes. If they do resent it, it is likely they just resent their diabetes.

continued

There will be other issues around their diabetes, how they are treated by family or friends, but the actual cause of having diabetes, most know, is not anything you have done.

Getting into a routine, including one for injections, will help make it part of your child's daily life. For example, in the morning and evening we do our teeth and before meals we do our injection; except of course they are the only ones who have to do an injection. Even young children will be aware of this difference.

Children learn by copying other people's behaviour. As parents, you are their role models. Perhaps doing a 'dry shot' injection with them on yourself will help them see that it is not a punishment and that it doesn't have to be a big deal. If they see you doing an injection, or you allow your child to inject you and see you are not scared they will be less likely to be scared, until they are old enough to have it all explained (see **What you can do** at the end of the chapter).

You might well be scared about having an injection yourself. Is your son picking up on your fear? Memories of injections are usually associated with pain. Most children and adults will have had vaccinations and many of them are painful, in part because vaccinations need to be given into a muscle, which hurts, using a special needle that is quite long and wide. Insulin injections are into the fat under the skin, which requires much smaller and thinner needles. If done with a good technique, insulin injections don't need to hurt. For little children, it can be more distressing to be restrained than to have the injection, so give some thought to how you hold him.

Doing an injection yourself without insulin is commendable but be careful not to gloat (See what I did!). Try and put yourself in their shoes; consider doing injections and blood tests when your child does for a whole week and then reread this book.

They think I'm amazing and say, 'I don't know how you can do that'. I think, it's not like I've got any choice.
(Amanda, 9)

When I first saw the injection I ran away from it. I was just scared. They had to calm me down. They said 'I'll try not to make it hurt'. It did hurt me when I was that age. When I was six I got used to it because I was having it so often. Now sometimes it might hurt for a few seconds, that's it.

(Jeffrey, 9)

Q Is it better to let my child miss an injection and feel unwell, or force her into it?

A This is a tricky one. High blood glucose levels, as well as some low ones, are a normal part of having diabetes. Both will occur and might be unavoidable. So long as either highs or lows occur for only brief periods, they are unlikely to do any real harm, provided that your child does not develop ketones. Hyperglycaemia on its own may make your child feel lethargic, tired and thirsty or she may not notice any symptoms at all.

Your child needs to know the consequences of their own actions since she will eventually need to take ownership of her diabetes in order to live an independent life. Ignoring injections will ultimately spoil this independence; running high glucose levels or swinging from high to low will make her feel unwell, affect her mood and behaviour and may even result eventually in diabetic complications (see Chapter 6: Hyperglycaemia, ketoacidosis and complications).

Your child will know better than you what it feels like to run high. Try to help her realise that this is related to whether she takes her injection or not. It can be an empowering time for a young person to realise there are consequences to their actions and that their behaviour can affect how they feel. Diabetes is an incredibly powerful button that can easily be pressed to self-destruct as an act of rebellion. The young person gains this means of control, not only of their diabetes, but also of you: it can sometimes be used as a tool to manipulate parents.

Why should I have to do an injection? Even if I know someone else also has to do an injection it still feels like I am the only one who has to have it done.

(Janina, 13)

Q Gary is eight and developing lumps in his tummy. I have been told to rotate sites but he refuses to try any others and his tummy is the only place he will do his injections. What can I do?

A Allow your child time; no one likes to be pressured. He may be scared that a new site is going to hurt more. Often other children who are in the same position are the only ones that will convince your child to try somewhere new and are usually willing to show others, more scared, how to do it.

Learning to inject a new site for the first time can be as scary as leaning how to do an injection for the first time. The skin is more sensitive, you need to learn a new technique, and your child may not want to leave injection marks elsewhere.

You may think, 'What's the big deal? An injection is an injection' and you'd be wrong. All those with diabetes will have their favourite site, which may be related to pain levels or sites that can be conveniently reached. There is no 'right time' for a child, or adult, to learn to inject a new site. Pushing them into it can create a new battle and make them dig in their heels even more. It can also make them feel frightened and vulnerable.

You may need to go back to the routine you went through when learning how to inject for the first time. Practise on teddies, then on yourself, and then mimic injecting at the new site before a needle goes anywhere near.

It is important to help Gary understand why he needs to change sites. After all, what's the point of changing sites for no reason? Choose a time to talk about it that's not around injection time. Try to ask him why he doesn't want to try a new site. It might be enough to introduce the idea little by little, allowing him time to

continued on next page

A *continued*

digest the information and in his own time decide when it is the right time.

Talking through the issues and trying to let your child come up with the idea of changing injection sites for themselves is more likely to bring positive results. Introduce new information slowly – small building blocks soon grow into towers of strength.

I tried my bum once but I got cramp. I don't do my legs – it hurts more.

(Janina, 13)

Sometimes I feel like I've run out of sites.

(Mike, 27)

I had lumps and kept doing them in the lumps. After that I was going high and then going low. I went on a diabetic holiday and someone did a new site for me.

(Kaya, 12)

I used to have lumps in my arms and my legs. Once I changed sites the lumps went down.

(Chantelle, 12)

I've done about ten injections on my own but always in my left arm. I got used to doing my injection in the same place. I got scared of injecting somewhere else.

(Liam, 12)

Q There is always an argument around injection time. My son often refuses to inject himself and it's always me rather than my husband who ends up doing it. I don't want my son to have to do an injection either, but I know he has to. How can we stop the arguments?

A Your child may just need some time. However, you also do not want it to become 'normal' to have to persuade your child to inject every time, or have a big argument. Talk to your diabetes team, who will have seen this before and will have some ideas about what to do. Talk with your son about it, but choose a time that is not near injection time. You could say something like this:

> ❝ I love you very much and wish you didn't have diabetes and need to take an injection. But you do. I don't like having to make you do your injection each time as I know it makes you sad, which also makes me sad. But I also know that you won't feel well if you don't have your injection.
> So what do you think we should do?
> How about we decide to wait a certain amount of time (say, for 15 minutes) and if you haven't started doing your injection by then we will go to the hospital and they will do it or I could do it here for you. ❞

Once you have agreed a rule, stick to it.

Sometimes it ends up that one parent gives most of the diabetes care. This is certainly the case for single parents. Diabetes can seem like a constant stress with little reward, just avoiding recurrent disasters. It seems unjust and you will ask yourself, 'Why should my child go through all this?'

If the routine isn't working for you as a family, both parents need to start sharing the load. If your other half isn't used to being part

continued on next page

of diabetes care they may make a mistake – like giving the wrong amount of insulin or forgetting to bring a snack along after school. Making them feel guilty will make them scared of getting involved with the diabetes any more. Your child will also pick up on it.

If there is always an argument at injection time, then try to take away any threats you may be making. There is no point having a confrontation; your son doesn't want to inject and you don't want him to have to, but he does. It is not the fault of either of you and creating an argument isn't doing anyone any good.

I used to have a phobia of needles but I managed to get on top of it as I got older and took things over. I went to diabetic camp. It really helped – they showed me how to inject my bum. Now it's not a big thing.

(Daniel, 17)

What you can do

- **Ask your child what would help.** It might be more time, some quiet, a private place to inject, practise, or even handing back the responsibility to you for a while to give them a break. Every child, and adult, needs personal space, irrespective of whether they have diabetes or not. Diabetes involves the body and so a need for privacy and space is even more important.

- **A 'dry shot'.** You will need to get your diabetes team to show you what this is and how to do it. Essentially it involves injecting without any liquid. You can use a pen device to mimic injecting insulin, making sure it's an unused needle. It is important that you do not inject any insulin because (if you do not have diabetes yourself) you could go hypo and may even become unconscious. You could get your child to inject you and also try injecting yourself. You will feel how scary it is putting the needle through your skin. You will also feel that it hurts far less than you thought it would.

- **Practise first** on an orange, then on a doll or teddy, then on yourself, and then let your child inject you. Break down the injection routine into a series of very small steps. Encourage your child to take part in one new step every few weeks, or when they are ready.
- **Learn through play in a safe environment.** Some hospitals have Play therapists who can help by introducing injecting as part of a diabetes routine through play. This is especially useful for younger children.
- **Keep home as a safe place.** If your child won't do their injection or won't let you do it for them don't force them. The last resort would be to give your child a set time, such as 15 minutes and then take them to the hospital. Discuss with your diabetes team any technique you could use.
- **Allow time.** If your child says they want time, give them it.
- **Ensure consistency** between you and your partner.

Injections

The first injection was all done,
But I didn't think it was much fun,
They said I needed to do it in the leg,
So I pulled up my trouser and tied it with a peg.

They pulled out the needle and I thought to myself:
This if for the good of my health,
"Here we go", the nurse did say,
"You can sit or you can lay."

I did not move, I sat there still,
Asking myself why I couldn't have a pill,
I squeezed my mum and dads arm,
Trying not to tense and be very calm.

I did it in the end and it wasn't very bad,
So there is no reason to be so sad.

Anna, 13, on injections

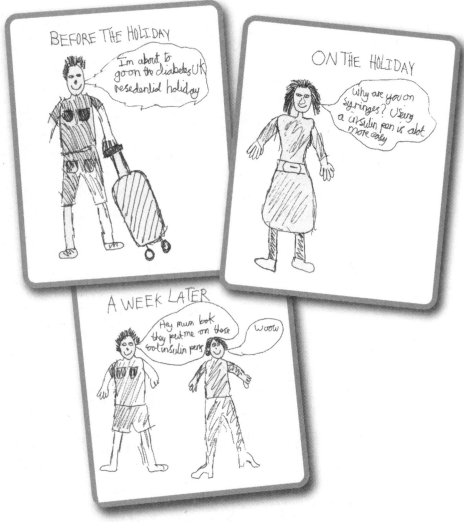

Children learn lots about injections at diabetes camp.

Rachel's view

It can be pretty boring hearing the same old comments about injections. Play another record, heard that one before! People wonder how I can inject myself. The answer is simple: because I have to. For me injections aren't the problem, the annoyance comes with the inconvenience and rules surrounding injections, as well the unwanted attention it brings. That's probably why I always injected in private when I was growing up unless I was with people who knew I had diabetes and didn't make an issue out of it. It's great going on diabetes camps; we all do our injections in front of each other. In fact it was at a camp when I was there as a volunteer before I became a doctor, when I was about 21, that a 10-year-old boy showed me how to inject my bottom for the first time. I was helping out in the injection room and a girl said she had never injected her bottom before. This boy said, 'It's easy' and showed us. I confessed that I had never injected my bum before either, as I hadn't liked the idea of it. He talked me through it and I did it. Well, I couldn't lose face! That night at dinner, he stood on a chair and announced to everyone that I had injected my bum for the first time. I had to stand up and take a bow. Thanks to him, I started injecting my bum and still do. It just shows that you are never too old to try a new site.

I think it's ridiculous if children aren't allowed to inject at the dinner table at school and are sent to the Medical Room instead. It's an unnecessary waste of time and reinforces the idea that children with diabetes are different. Sure, if they want to do it in private then they should be allowed. If not, I don't understand what the fuss is all about. Children with inhalers use them in the classroom.

I used to inject at table when out with my family but my brother used to worry that other people minded. Perhaps he just didn't like watching his little sister doing an injection and thought it hurt me. I've never let anyone do my injection after I was first diagnosed. It's much easier to do injections for yourself. You can tell when it hurts and then you stop and reposition.

Now I am on an insulin pump. It is less of a hassle because of the physiology of how the pump works rather than because of having to do fewer injections. When I went on my pump, after 14 years of injecting with syringes and pens, I missed the routine of the injections. When I did have to give an occasional injection, I enjoyed it.

My insulin pump is often obvious to other people. Many confuse it with a pager, and think I am continuously on call, or think I am permanently attached to my mobile phone. Some people recognise it and ask, 'Are you diabetic?' as if they are surprised that I am.

The pump needle is longer and does hurt sometimes, whereas I find that normal injections don't really hurt at all. However, having a pump has transformed my busy life.

Food and eating

What are the different constituents of food, and which ones affect blood glucose levels?

Our food is made up of:

■ carbohydrate;

■ protein;

■ fat;

■ vitamins and minerals.

All are needed for the body to function normally, to grow and develop.

Any food containing *carbohydrate* will raise blood glucose. Carbohydrates are food types which are made up of sugar molecules. They can be in a 'simple' form, which taste sweet and once eaten can be released quickly into the bloodstream, or molecules of sugar stacked together, termed *complex carbohydrates*. These foods, such as bread and potato, do not taste sweet and need to be broken down into their 'simple' forms before the sugar can be released into the bloodstream and raise the blood glucose level. Simple sugars get into the bloodstream and raise blood glucose levels faster but also leave the bloodstream faster than the complex carbohydrates.

Protein comes from fish, meat, eggs, pulses, nuts and seeds, soya and dairy products. Protein on its own does not raise blood glucose.

Fat, including oil, is found in many foods, both animal and vegetable. There are 'good' (unsaturated) and 'bad' (saturated or trans) fats. Fats do not contain carbohydrate but do affect how quickly carbohydrate-containing food reaches the bloodstream.

Vitamins and minerals are nutrients found mostly in fruit and vegetables. Whilst food containing vitamins and minerals may also contain carbohydrate, on their own they do not raise blood glucose levels.

What is carbohydrate counting?

People with diabetes need to match the carbohydrate they eat with insulin. Counting the carbohydrate in food gives you information so you can:

■ adjust the insulin dose to match the size of your meal;

■ eat meals with roughly the same carbohydrate content each day.

On a mixed-insulin regimen, there is less flexibility with adjusting insulin doses according to what you eat. Eating roughly the same amount of carbohydrate at each meal on mixed-insulin regimens is better for blood glucose stability. However, basal bolus (4 or 5-times-a-day) regimens and insulin pumps are perfectly suited to exact carbohydrate counting. This involves knowing the carbohydrate content of food, often in grams, and adjusting the amount of rapid-acting insulin accordingly.

How you actually do this involves learning about carbohydrates and some trial and error. A good place to start is to talk about the types of food your family likes to eat with your dietitian, who will show you easy ways of carbohydrate counting looking at portion sizes and using food tables and food labels. On a food label, the figure you need is under 'Total Carbohydrates' (rather than 'available' or 'other' carbohydrate or the carbohydrate 'of which sugars').

Carbohydrate counting can be simple: eyeballing food and deciding whether the carbohydrate it contains needs to be balanced with more or less insulin, or quite sophisticated, counting carbohydrates in grams. You will find the method that suits you. At first, eating out may be harder, but treat these times as experiments and don't worry too much: you can always give some more short-acting insulin when you get home if you need to.

The amount of insulin needed to balance the carbohydrate eaten (the insulin-to-carbohydrate ratio) varies between individuals and sometimes between different times of day. For example, an apple containing 15 g carbohydrate would not need the same amount of insulin in three individuals: one might need 1 unit of rapid-acting insulin, another may need 1.5, and another, on an insulin pump who can fine-tune insulin delivery even more, may need 0.8 units.

Most people find that the effort of learning how to carbohydrate count pays off: they now have more freedom to eat what and when they want.

We have seen that different types of carbohydrate raise blood glucose levels at different rates. This means that when you assess the carbohydrate in food, it is worth understanding how different carbohydrates do this. This is where the Glycaemic Index (GI) comes in.

What is the Glycaemic Index (GI)?

It is a way of measuring how quickly a food will raise your blood glucose level. Foods with a higher GI increase blood glucose more quickly than those with a lower GI. The GI of a food is affected by several factors:

- the type of carbohydrate (for example, rice has a lower GI than potato);
- the amount of fibre (roughage);
- the amount of fat;
- the presence of a coating around the outside of a fruit or pulse (all of which decrease GI);
- method of food preparation and cooking;
- the amount of liquid and salt within the food (all of which raise the GI).

This means that food with a lower GI, such as porridge oats, will cause a slower rise in blood glucose levels and will be available for longer than Puffed Wheat with a high GI. You can delay the release of glucose from sweeter foods into the bloodstream by eating them at the end of a meal, particularly one with a higher fat content.

What are the best foods for people with diabetes?

Everyone should be eating a healthy balanced diet, whether they have diabetes or not. This means a healthy balance of carbohydrate, protein, fat, fibre, vitamins, minerals and salt.

Food marketed as 'diabetic' is not recommended; these often have more fat in than their non-diabetic counterparts, and use artificial sweeteners which can cause stomach problems and diarrhoea if eaten in excess; also, they are usually expensive. You can incorporate small amounts of ordinary sweet foods into meals and snacks, so long as they are balanced with adequate insulin and levels of physical activity.

Most people eat far too much fat; not only does it cause weight gain, but also in the longer term increases the risk of atherosclerosis (blocked arteries) and heart disease. Poor glucose control on its own can lead to atherosclerosis and heart disease, so a high fat diet increases this risk even further. Those with diabetes often gain more weight than those of the same age without diabetes, so weight management is important.

A low-salt diet is recommended to reduce high blood pressure which can contribute to diabetic complications.

Is there anything you can't eat if you have diabetes?

No, nothing is banned. People with diabetes can eat the same food as other people, so long as any carbohydrate food is balanced with insulin.

What is coeliac disease and who is affected?

Coeliac disease is caused by an intolerance to the protein gluten that is present in wheat, rye, barley and some oats. It occurs in up to 10% of children with diabetes. If someone with coeliac disease eats gluten it may cause tummy problems such as stomach pain, constipation and diarrhoea; it may also cause delayed growth or puberty, poor nutrition and hypoglycaemia. Like diabetes, coeliac is an autoimmune condition (see Chapter 1). See the Appendix for more information and sources of support on coeliac disease.

Are eating disorders more common in diabetes?

Eating disorders, which range in severity, are relatively common in people with diabetes, especially young women. Causes of eating disorders are complex. Much of the focus of diabetes management is around food, and so perhaps it is not surprising that eating disorders occur more often in people with diabetes than in those without. If you have diabetes and do not take insulin it will cause weight loss, regardless of what you eat, because without insulin, protein and fat are broken down; ketones accumulate and there is the inevitable hyperglycaemia. The ketones make the blood acidic and cause nausea and, if untreated, vomiting, as well as reducing appetite. If insulin is not given when ketones are present, an individual can become ill very quickly with diabetic ketoacidosis (see Chapter 6).

Introduction to the cases

Case studies do not usually need an introduction, but a warning is needed here because you may find these personal stories disturbing. They are an honest look at what some young people with eating disorders may experience, and include descriptions of dangerous behaviours in handling food and insulin. We need to understand why people find themselves in this position, and this is what I attempt in the discussion later on. These are extreme cases, but I suspect that experiences such as these, some less serious and some even more, may be commoner than people realise.

Case 1

A young woman talks about bulimia

Introducing Martina, 28, diagnosed aged 7

Your life's so focused on food and weight, when something's wrong it's the easiest thing to control. You can tell people what you can and can't eat. You start to have one chocolate bar, realise it doesn't kill you and so starts the slippery slope.

When anything goes wrong in your life you start to relate it to food and diabetes.

At school when I was about 15, other girls were smoking and skipping meals. I was aware I had to eat loads 'cos of my diabetes. It made me feel greedy but actually I was eating what a non-diabetic should eat. You do things to make yourself feel better and I'd do anything to stop myself thinking about food. Smoking would suppress my appetite and so would ketones.

I was put on a different insulin regime to give me more freedom. I could have more freedom, less insulin and less food. I started to lose weight healthily. But I didn't stop, I got obsessed with it. But with diabetes you have hypos and you have to eat. One day I had a hypo, ate some fudge and couldn't stop eating. I ate everything in sight. I tried to give an injection for it and spent the next week exercising to make up for it. My sugars were all over the shop. I tried using laxatives and slimming pills. It became a cycle of diet, binge, exercise.

I approached my clinic to say I had a problem. The diabetic nurse

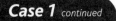

Case 1 *continued*

said that it's not uncommon to see eating disorders with diabetes and that she knew of one girl with DKA (diabetic ketoacidosis) who wasn't injecting herself to lose weight. It was like, 'Why didn't I think of that!' So I didn't inject after binges after that. I found that I not only didn't put on weight but I lost it. It got to the point that I wouldn't inject the day after a binge, the day after that and then the day after that. I cut down my insulin, only doing background insulin every couple of days. I lost a lot of weight. I was a dead person walking. I somehow managed so I didn't go into a coma. I think I had a Guardian Angel.

When I was about 17, the turning point came at work. I sat on a seat. I looked at the floor and thought, if I shut my eyes I'm going to go into a coma and die.

The hospital had told me that if I didn't start injecting myself and stop smoking I'd die. I was just a number to them. My doctor wanted to help me but I moved from adolescent to adult clinic and I never saw him again. In clinic I was a teenager with all these 40-year-olds.

In adult clinic I saw a different doctor every time and they didn't know me on a personal basis, they just knew me as a number. They saw a diabetic teenager who wasn't looking after themselves. Actually I needed deep emotional help, not them just telling me I would die.

'We can't do anything for you until you start injecting', they'd say.

I went to my GP and said I needed help. It was only my GP who referred me to a psychiatrist. After a while the psychiatrist said, 'We've done everything we can, on your way'. I went out, binged and didn't inject myself for a few days. I went back to my GP again who referred me to a psychologist. With her help I was able to detangle the web of emotion I had tangled myself up in, rebuild my relationship with diabetes first and then with food. I had a relapse a year after, for a year, then got back on track.

I still haven't talked about it with my family, even now. I think they thought it was just that I wasn't looking after my diabetes properly. I don't think they knew that I had an eating disorder or that my diabetes was tangled up in an eating disorder.

continued on next page

Case 1 *continued*

Even now I have a good relationship with food but it takes a stronger presence than it should. I have to be aware and on guard when it is. You're never free of an eating disorder. With diabetes you feel like it controls you. If you can control it you can feel powerful.

A young woman talks about anorexia

Introducing Ruth, 38, diagnosed aged 14

When they first said I was diabetic it wasn't me, it was something outside me that I had to fit into. I felt totally wrong. Mum was over-fussy. There was so much I wasn't allowed to do. My life wasn't my own. Everyone had a say in what I did and what I ate except me. Everyone knew better. There was this mould that I had to fit into. Mum didn't think I had a say in it, as I was a child, she thought she was helping. She felt so guilty and felt my life would be made easier if she took it all over from me. It was this burden she wanted to take away. But it became very controlling. Even now Mum says, 'What do you mean you haven't eaten yet?' I'm 38!

Food was always a big issue in our house, even before the diabetes. I was rebelling at that age anyway. Mum controlled all my eating. She used to prepare my lunch box and I'd chuck it away.

I had started to put on some weight with all the snacks and every time I did sport I had to eat. I went to the doctor but he said I was fine and he wouldn't help me take control of my weight gain. I was stood there thinking, 'I do have a problem'. I thought, no one will help me and Mum kept giving me food. I decided to deal with it myself. I started throwing food away but because I was still injecting I started having big hypos and passing out. Then I suddenly realised, if I didn't take my insulin I wouldn't have a hypo.

As I became obsessive it started to get out of hand. I was trying to regain control but I was losing control. It was never about being thin. At first I didn't feel ill when my blood was high. Then I started to feel sick so I didn't feel hungry either. Everything rolled out of control and it continued until I was 26.

At first no one noticed. I used to fill my pockets full of money when I was weighed at the clinic. I was admitted to hospital for various reasons related to my eating. Looking back, they knew it was to do with my diabetes but no one talked to me about it. All they said was, 'You have to keep your blood sugars better controlled'.

Eventually when I was 18 I was taken away to live in a home. I was admitted for my eating disorder, not because of my diabetes. The diabetes was ignored. If they made me eat I threw up. It became a game. I thought, whatever you do, I'll beat you. I focused on that rather than anything else. I thought if I messed up my diabetes enough I could make myself small enough and disappear, then I wouldn't be a problem to anyone. I thought that because of my diabetes everyone had focused on me. I felt guilty about everything – my brother didn't have enough attention, arguments between Mum and Dad, I felt it was all my fault. I kept everyone at arm's length. It was easier that way; otherwise they'd become part of my eating. I wasn't going to share my life with anyone.

I kept my weight on the brink of near admission and injected enough to keep me out of hospital. Then I started doing a night class and realised that I loved designing and I had found something for me. I thought, I want to live again.

I went to university. My eating wasn't right and I was so thin. I used to wear layers of jumpers. Then the turning point came when I was 27 and was admitted to hospital for 6 months with a diabetes-related problem. I was transferred to a hospital and for the first time they listened.

Discussion

Martina and Ruth in Case 1 developed severe eating disorders, bulimia in the case of Martina and anorexia in Ruth's. It is unclear whether or not they would have developed the eating disorders if they hadn't had diabetes. What is striking is the way they both used their diabetes as a tool to empower them in their eating. Diabetes is unique in that it can be manipulated; by withholding insulin, you can actively lose weight without even having to eat less food. This is dangerous: by omitting insulin, high blood glucose levels accumulate, fat and protein are broken down in the body and ketones are produced, which will also take away appetite.

Clearly other influences were at play in both cases, such as peer pressure to be thin in the case of Martina, and Ruth's feeling of loss of control. In both cases, diabetes became the focus: food was an easy thing to control and insulin easy to manipulate. Ruth's mother had bulimia and a complex relationship with food. Ruth felt that she, and her food intake, was being controlled by her mother. It is unclear whether her mother was over-controlling subconsciously, in her desire to 'just follow the rules', or whether her own difficulties around Ruth's diagnosis and her own eating behaviour was influencing her interaction with Ruth.

Many people with diabetes are told what they can and cannot eat. Once they realise that actually they can break the rules and get away with it in the short term, food becomes the focus of an easy act of rebellion. Unfortunately the message itself is false, as things have changed. Not so long ago, diabetes was managed by strict carbohydrate counting and portion sizes; the insulins available were not sophisticated and needed to be injected 30 minutes before eating. Food was then eaten at specific times of the day, and what could be eaten was a certain portion size or amount of carbohydrate. The portions, also called exchanges, were measured using scales or estimated using standard measures, such as a template grid to count bread portions and egg sizes to count rice or potato portions. Meals and snacks had to be eaten at certain times of the day, with an exact amount of carbohydrate, as a portion or in grams, irrespective of how hungry you were. There were other rules, such as no sweet foods. This is different now. Current diabetes diets should be a 'normal healthy diet', and one which everyone should follow, whether they have diabetes or not. The newer insulins also allow for adjustments with exercise, so that large snacks may not be necessary, although this depends on the type and duration of exercise, the insulin and the individual. This is discussed in more detail in Chapter 3. The younger child who has two injections per day still has to observe some rigidity around meal and snack times. However, as discussed in Chapter 4, the introduction of newer insulin regimens has brought more flexibility with food. Realistically, though, it is difficult not to have rules about food with diabetes, although they are more relaxed these days.

Most people who are not part of the diabetes community, and even those who are, still have the idea that to have diabetes means you cannot eat certain foods. This misconception is transferred to children and their families, and causes confusion. It brings annoyance, resentment and a feeling of being different. Someone acting in the best interests of a child may deliberately not offer that child a biscuit or slice of cake. Think how annoyed and resentful that would make you feel! With some education and balancing, these problems can be solved, but it all may seem such an effort.

Having said all that, as a parent you will know that sweeter foods do raise blood glucose levels more than savoury ones. You may feel that cutting out all sweet foods will help diabetes control, and you are right, of course. But anyone who has ever tried to stick to a diet will know how hard it is. Try doing it forever, and you will understand that it is near impossible without some misery.

Many children who were brought up on the old, stricter regimens, who are now young adults, will talk about cheating and hiding foods. This will happen anyway, so surely it is better not to go through the pretence and to allow some sweet foods, within reason, to be included every day?

Martina and Ruth were both brought up on the old-fashioned diabetic diet. It would be too easy to blame this entirely for their eating disorders. It certainly gave them powerful tools to seize control which others do not have at their disposal: missing injections causing hyperglycaemia and ketoacidosis, suppressing appetite and avoiding hypos. Even on current regimens and dietary advice, food can still be made a big issue with or without diabetes. Eating disorders, or unhealthy relationships with food, are probably a lot more common than is realised.

Martina remembers clearly a hypo as the initial trigger for the start of her bulimia. Many people, as discussed in Chapter 2, get a sort of food rage in response to their hypo. It is the body's way of saying, 'Hey, I need some sugar, quick!' It is different from the feeling one gets with hunger, but something like it. Hunger is often an unreliable sign of having a hypo, compared to other feelings such as tiredness. However, children may say they feel 'hungry' when they are hypo as a way of communicating that they need food. Having diabetes means having hypos which need to be treated with food. This starts a reinforcing pattern of behaviour of eating when you are not hungry. Food is eaten in response to hypos, at certain times of the day and before exercise. It is easy for food to become something that is tied up to an emotion rather than hunger.

Case 2

Balancing food intake against blood glucose levels

Introducing Jeffrey, 9, diagnosed aged 4

If your blood is 12 you shouldn't really have something to eat. If you're hungry you should eat something small like a yoghurt. If I know what my sugar level is and I'm not allowed to eat it I might have one chocolate and leave it for a bit. Sometimes I want to have more 'cos it's really nice. Sometimes I think I might want it and my sugar level's too high. If I'm high I won't be able to have anything to eat. I might want to go to the toilet a lot and be rushing around.

I check my blood sugar and I might have it [the chocolate] if I think it is good enough – 7 or 8. If I'm 10 I might have a little bit of what it is. If I'm 8 I might have nearly all of it.

Discussion

Even Jeffrey, who is only 9 and since diagnosis at age 4 has been brought up on today's modern diabetes regimen, still talks as if he is a number and being 'good enough', implying a degree of failure if his blood glucose is high. To some degree he has a very advanced level of understanding about what he should and shouldn't eat, based on his blood glucose level. However, he is also reinforcing his own pattern of behaviour, which is deciding what and when to eat because of a number, rather than the 'normal' way, which is 'Do I like that food? Do I want to eat it? Am I hungry?' He could have the chocolate and some extra insulin.

Some of these behaviours are unavoidable. You need to talk with your child and think about what they say; this is a good opportunity to challenge their way of thinking and be sure they are keeping that healthy relationship with you, their diabetes and with food. If you don't ask your child how they feel, however, you will never know.

Q How can I avoid making food a big deal?

A Food does not have to become a big deal but it is an easy thing to focus on if you have diabetes. Much of what gives children food

continued

issues is how other people react and what they say to them. This will be based on others' perception of diabetes. Their perceptions will often be based on the way diabetes used to be managed. Not that long ago diabetes was managed with old-fashioned, inflexible insulin which had to be given half an hour before eating; food was eaten at set times and with strict portion sizes. It is easy to see how food became a big issue. Even today, depending on attitude and personal experience, food can still be at the centre of your child's diabetes and will affect what you and others tell your child about what they can and cannot eat. Some of this will depend on how much information you are given, and partly on what type of insulin your child is on. It is important that you have a healthy attitude to food yourself and the way you teach your child about how it interplays with their diabetes so that they can learn to live a healthy life, both in mind and body.

Food is an essential part in anyone's life, with or without diabetes. Anyone who has ever been on, or tried to go on, a diet will know that diets are hard. A life-long diet would be near impossible to stick to, but this is how diabetes used to be managed. These days, a diabetes diet is said to be a 'normal healthy diet'. Whilst this is true, and encourages those with diabetes to eat the same as everybody else, we know that not everyone does eat healthily. Ultimately, having high-sugar foods a lot of the time is going to raise and cause swings in blood glucose levels.

Children often feel that with diabetes the choice has been taken away from them. Even if they know they might not want to eat five bowls of ice-cream, the fact that they are not supposed to seems unfair. In fact they can eat it, but they may feel rather unwell if not enough insulin is given.

It is recommended that you check blood glucose levels only 1½–2 hours after eating because of the inevitable hyperglycaemia that follows eating carbohydrate-containing food. If this is inappropriately corrected it may cause hypoglycaemia. The trouble is that 2 hours after eating, most people are eating again, because the current trend in eating habits is constant 'grazing'. This can cause chronic raised blood glucose levels all day, except for people with diabetes who use

continued on next page

an insulin pump and can give a bolus of insulin through the pump whenever food is eaten, without doing an injection.

Healthy eating is not just about choosing healthy foods, it is about when and how you eat. Eating meals at the table with appropriate small snacks between meals encourages healthy eating behaviour and also helps blood glucose control. However, most young people like junk food. Often this is the type of food that contains carbohydrate that is absorbed quickly into the blood and contains junk such as salt and lots of fat, both of which in the long term promote changes which contribute to development of complications, such as raised blood pressure and heart disease (see Chapter 6).

Developing early healthy attitudes to food is important for yourself and your family; good habits will rub off on your child. Many children are incorrectly told that they are not allowed to eat sweets, particularly around the time of diagnosis. This is what often sticks out in their minds, rather than the fear of injections, repeated blood testing and complications. It is important that your child can understand about food when they are old enough. Until then, it is every parent's responsibility to give their child healthy food choices as these are usually the types of foods that children will go on to choose for themselves when they are in a position to do so. After all, we are what we eat.

The one thing I could control was food.

(Martina, 28)

I eat the same sort of snacks that they do in school.

(Kaya, 12)

When I was younger I couldn't eat sweets - it made it a bigger deal. Sometimes I got annoyed and buy sweets.

(Janina, 13)

At the beginning I couldn't eat anything. They made me cry at the hospital, saying I could never eat a jam doughnut again, that really upset me. School always acted inappropriately through lack of knowledge. On Cake Day, I wouldn't get any and I was really pissed off. Mum understood about diabetes, she got it and just changed my insulin depending on what I was eating.

(Jason, 27)

I eat less chocolate bars now than before I was diagnosed but I still eat chocolate after school. I'll give extra insulin.

(Luke, 17)

I never used to eat a lot of sweets so that's not a problem but having to inject every time you eat gets a little bit boring.

(Liam, 12)

Q **Cake Day at school, Easter, Halloween and birthday parties are difficult times. Is it better to offer my child sweets, cakes and biscuits and let them decide, or ask for them not to be offered any at all?**

A Not being offered food at parties or being offered it with a back-hander, like 'you're not allowed to eat that, are you?', makes children with diabetes feel different. As discussed in previous chapters, feeling different is a major issue with childhood diabetes and can lead to a feeling of isolation and resentment. Whilst you may be focusing on your child's blood glucose reading, they will be wondering whether the Pass-the-Parcel will land with them or how late they will be allowed to stay up at the sleepover. The last thing on your child's mind will be their diabetes. Quite right too, you want them to enjoy their childhood with all the fun it can bring. They may well take what is offered to them and then their blood glucose will rise.

This is the time to talk about why their blood glucose is high, and

continued on next page

what you could do at the next party: perhaps giving a little more insulin at mealtime or correcting with some rapid-acting insulin in the middle or at the end of the party. It will depend on your child's insulin regimen and how much activity there will be at the party: lots of running about or a bouncy castle will bring down blood glucose, and cake will raise it.

However, the party may be a one-off or your child may not be on the type of insulin regimen that allows for a bit of extra rapid-acting insulin to cover for a hungry or sweet-tooth moment. You may need to correct their blood glucose later with some extra insulin. Perhaps they can eat some of the sweets and keep the rest for later, such as instead of a snack, or at the end of a meal for pudding.

There is a fine balance to be struck here. On the one hand you do not want your child's blood glucose swinging all over the place all the time, but on the other hand you do not want your child to be treated differently or to feel different.

It is often up to you as a parent to educate other people who deal with your child. Remember that although diabetes management has changed radically over the past 20 years, people's perception of it has not. Don't let other people's lack of knowledge affect your child's fun and fulfilment in life.

When I was little I used to eat loads of sweets 'cos they're so delicious. Now I only eat a couple at a time. I understand more – you need to control your blood sugars.

(Margaret, 12)

We were strict at first, avoiding sugary things. Such a big deal was made about food. Food controlled you and was a way of fighting back. I hate it when people say, 'You're not allowed to eat that'. I know what I can and can't do. What's going to happen – is the world going to end? I've learnt when they are passing cake around at work to say no and restrain myself.

(Mike, 27)

At work it would be nice to be offered and say, 'No, thanks', otherwise the person who didn't know I had diabetes will ask me later why I couldn't eat it, I'll feel awkward about it and worry about what they think.

(Ruth, 38)

I hate people who say, 'Ooooooh you're not meant to eat that are you dear?', when they see you eat chocolate or a bit of cake and at these times I wish people would be a bit more clued up and let me get on with my diabetes. How do they know that I didn't check my sugars and they were 4 mmols and I could feel myself dropping so I had some nice cake OR (shock, horror) I JUST FANCIED SOME and gave myself a little extra shot of insulin?

(Juliet, 22)

I try and stop myself eating sweets. I get cravings at the end of the day if my bloods are down and I have to eat there and then. I can eat popcorn, two chocolate bars and a bottle of coke. I think it's a rebellion thing. People tell you that you can't eat sweets. My friends can eat it whenever they want. If I go to my cousin's house, he's close to me like my brother. He understands my cravings and Mum nagging me all the time. He offers me food and says, 'Take it only if you want it'. Certain people might offer me sweets. They're trying to be nice by asking me. I want it but it's not good for me. I think, if you know I shouldn't be eating it, don't offer it to me.

(Daniel, 17)

Q We don't have sugary foods in the house for my son who is 11 and has diabetes. I worry that my other son who doesn't have diabetes is being punished. Sometimes I buy him sweets and tell him not to let on. Is that OK?

A Little secrets, however well meaning, tend to slip out at some point. If you're lucky, this one may not, but I am still concerned that you are treating your children differently – and so are you. It will affect how your son who does not have diabetes feels about your son who does.

There is no reason that both your children can't have the same treats at the same time. If they don't, you are treating them differently and they may end up feeling different from each other and other boys their age. Perhaps you may feel that you are punishing your son who has diabetes. Even if you reassure yourself that you are giving him extra presents, it will not make up for seeing others having things he has been told he is not allowed.

I hate it when people say 'You're lucky because you have to eat'. I think, I'd swap places with you.

(George, 35)

Q Recently I found sweet packets hidden in Tina's room. It may explain some recent high blood sugars. Should I tell her off?

A Would you tell her off if she didn't have diabetes? If you would, then do. Remember that it is not Tina's fault she has diabetes. You are asking and expecting her to follow certain rules. You might be better off asking yourself why your daughter has eaten sweets and why she has felt the need to hide the evidence. Is she rebelling? Does she think she will get told off? Is she seeking attention from you by making her blood sugars high, or hoping that you will find the sweet wrappers?

Your child may not have even thought about eating sweets except when she was told that she shouldn't be eating them. The natural reaction is to eat them. After all, what is the worst thing that'll

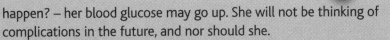

continued

happen? – her blood glucose may go up. She will not be thinking of complications in the future, and nor should she.

As discussed, there is no reason why sweet foods cannot be incorporated into everyday life or as part of a treat. It is much less likely to cause high blood glucose levels if it is thought about in advance.

when I was younger I used to pretend I was hypo so I could eat food. Now I just eat and give extra insulin.

(Katherine, 30)

I can't eat a lot of sweets, only before exercise. But you want to eat it badly, so I go to the shops, buy it and eat it. Sometimes they (my friends) think that if they eat sweets in front of me I'll be angry. I'm not really bothered – everywhere you go you see people eating sweets.

(Kiet, 16)

Sometimes my brother buys sweets and leaves them in the cupboard and I'll eat them but I don't like being thirsty. I'll take two bars of chocolate and then eat the whole lot and don't give an injection. I can't be bothered to get it out, dial it up and get the needle out.

(Janina, 13)

Q **Caroline has coeliac disease and diabetes. Many of the foods that are recommended for diabetes should be avoided with coeliac disease. Sometimes I feel we are all being punished twice. Does everyone feel like this? What are my options?**

A Many children with diabetes and coeliac disease find that having coeliac disease is the more challenging; it demands major changes in the diet, and in comparison diabetes is 'a doddle'. What makes it

continued on next page

A *continued*

particularly difficult is that many foods discouraged in coeliac disease commonly form the staple food in diabetes. It also adds a whole extra dimension to the food and diabetes equation, and often feels as though food choices are even more limited, on top of the limitations of diabetes. However, these days there is an ever-increasing availability of gluten-free foods which are suitable for those with coeliac disease, although many complain they are tasteless.

Luckily my son's diet was good so we didn't need to make any major changes - until a month later when they told us he also had coeliac disease. That was just too much because it really felt as though someone was having a joke at our expense. We had just reached the point when we could see some more flexibility on the horizon and suddenly all of that was taken away, so the two diagnoses seriously affected us all.

(A mother speaks about her 4-year-old)

It's quite balanced out because I have coeliac. I have to check the food labels. I'm used to it now.

(Margaret, 12)

I also have coeliac. Coeliac is worse than diabetes. At least with diabetes you can eat a little bit. Because I'm used to not eating sweets it's just another thing I can't eat. Seeing other people I'm envious they don't have to think about it. They can just go out and eat. Most of them [my friends] don't eat cakes when I'm there, and mum buys food free from stuff. My friends can eat anything they want. But your whole world doesn't revolve around food...at least I can still eat.

(Janina, 13)

What you can do

- **Ask how your child feels, and listen to what they say.** Ask how they would like to deal with a special situation, such as a party. Children need to feel listened to and are much more likely not to pretend about food behaviours if the plan of action comes from them.

- **All change!** The whole family needs to make adjustments together. Don't expect your child with diabetes to follow a different set of rules from you or your other children. That includes not sneaking a bar of chocolate to siblings when your child with diabetes is out of the house. Even if they won't find out about it, it will reinforce to siblings that they are different as they are being treated differently. Speak with your diabetes team about how to incorporate treats into meals and snacks.

- **Avoid temptations at home.** Don't leave sweets lying around the house if you don't want your child to eat them. At the same time, don't forget to have some pick-me-ups in the house to treat hypos – some Lucozade or glucose tablets and something that lasts a bit longer, like a cereal bar.

- **Learn through education.** One of the best ways of learning is to work things out for yourself. Playing learning games with groups of children can be fun; for example, working out how Easter eggs may affect blood glucose levels near Easter time by thinking about carbohydrates and looking at food packaging. Your dietitian or diabetes nurse may have their own games to help children think and come up with the answers themselves.

- **Explain the food ins and outs of diabetes to your child.** In doing so, you may find gaps in your own knowledge: after all, there has been a lot to take in. Ask your diabetes team for help.

Here is an example of how to explain to your child the issues surrounding food and how it affects blood glucose levels. You will need to adjust the words to suit your child. Try to avoid the phrase 'you can never eat sweets and chocolate again'. Most people with diabetes will have been told this, incorrectly, and it is easy for it to remain a bone of contention.

❦ With diabetes, the part of your body which produces insulin, which is called the pancreas, does not work properly. In someone who doesn't have diabetes, every time they eat food that contains sugar the body knows very quickly and releases insulin to bring the sugar level in their body down. It is very clever, so that insulin is released in exactly the right amount to bring the sugar in your blood to the right level, to feel healthy. In diabetes, the body cannot produce insulin on its own.

When I talk about sugar, I do not just mean things like chocolate and cakes. Sugar is in lots of other foods, even ones that don't taste sweet. These are foods like bread, rice, pasta and potatoes. When you eat those foods the body breaks them up into little bits in your tummy to produce sugar that goes into your blood and causes your blood sugar to rise. This can take several hours. This is why if you eat a bowl of sweets your blood sugar will go high very quickly, but if you eat a bowl of pasta the sugar from the pasta is broken down and released into your blood a lot more slowly. With diabetes, your body does not make insulin any more and so it can't work out how much insulin it needs to give at any one time. So, we will need to work it out. Some of what we decide to give will depend on how much food you eat and how much sugar is in the food. It sounds difficult but it's not really and just takes a bit of getting used to.

Eating some sweet foods, in someone with or without diabetes, is fine. But eating too many sugary foods, whether you have diabetes or not, is not a good thing. It can rot your teeth and make you put on weight. However, with diabetes we will need to think about how best to eat the sweet food so that it doesn't raise the blood sugar too much, otherwise you might not feel well.

Let's think of what we could do.

One thing would be to give a little bit of extra insulin.

Another would be to have it as part of your meal.

Another idea might be to save the treat until before PE (although the others at school might get jealous and it might make you look different to them).

What do you think would work best for you?

You can try all of them and see which suits you best. You might do one thing on one day and something else on another, or a combination.

Many people who don't understand diabetes will tell you that you can't eat sweet things. That is because they don't understand diabetes as well as you do and you might need to explain things to them. ⸾

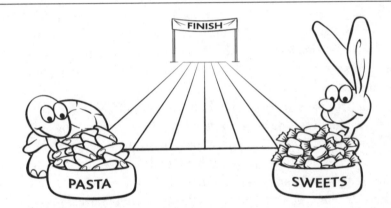

The bowl of sweets and the bowl of pasta contain the same amount of sugar.

Rachel's view

I was brought up at a time when you had to inject half-an-hour before eating and then make up the meal with a fixed amount of carbohydrate. It used to be 40 g for breakfast, 50 g for lunch and supper and 20 g for snacks in between meals and before bed. I would need to weigh some foods such as cereals to work out the carbohydrate value: food labels were not common, which made things more taxing. It didn't matter so much how that carbohydrate was made up, although there were other rules such as no sweets so inevitably it would be made up of potatoes or rice with fruit for pudding. There were other rules too, such as no salt, one egg and one bag of crisps a week, chips every so often and no fried food, only grilled. If I was hungry outside a meal or snack time I would eat non-carbohydrate food such as a piece of cold chicken, some soup or vegetables. On the one hand that sounds restrictive, but on the other I don't have any fillings, never went through the acne stage and growing up my blood sugars were very good.

As I got older the insulins became less rigid, and I changed from two to four injections a day. I seemed to miss seeing a dietitian for a few years after I was diagnosed, but I saw one again when I was about 14 who said that they didn't manage diabetes with strict carbohydrate rules any more, and that I could eat a 'normal healthy diet' and not count carbohydrates. I didn't know what she meant or how to do it. I felt guilty as I was still following the same rules and counting each gram of carbohydrate I ate as it had become part of my daily routine. I also felt guilty if I ate outside of the old rules. When I went to university I started to eat new foods but I didn't know how to incorporate it with my diabetes. I started eating sweet foods and felt guilty about it.

A year after I qualified as a doctor I went on an insulin pump and it was like being released from a lifetime's prison sentence. With my pump, suddenly I could do what the diabetes team pretend you can do – eat normally. It also gave me permission to count carbohydrates again, although I had never really stopped. Since I was diagnosed actual foods have changed: apples have got bigger – they used to be 10g and are now 15g – and slices of bread are thicker.

It is not just food that my pump has liberated me with. I work antisocial shifts and my life is busy, which means that I can't stop and eat at predictable times. My pump allows me to keep a steady amount of insulin going in the right amount to avoid big hypos and hypers. With a pump I felt better, as I was having fewer swings in blood glucose; I lost 8kg without even trying as I was having hypos which were less severe and didn't need to be fed. I can change my background basal rate, to allow a higher rate in the early hours of the morning and reduce the rate in the afternoon and before exercise. These variations are just not possible with any of the long-acting insulins currently available.

The old-fashioned restrictive carbohydrate rules of the 1980s could be followed with good blood glucose results. Even when this was relaxed, by switching to taking insulin before meals, it was still hard juggling food, insulin and a busy life. However, some of the newer long-acting insulin analogues, such as glargine and Levemir, which would have made life easier, were not around when I went on a pump. My HbA$_{1c}$ was always pretty good, but at the expense of a massive effort, which didn't leave a lot of room for everything else I wanted in my life.

Seven years on, my diabetes really does fit in with my life. I do what I want and eat what I want. I am a Specialist Registrar in acute paediatrics; two years ago I cycled through Vietnam and Cambodia (raising £4000 for Diabetes UK) and last year was the group medic on a trek along the Great Wall of China.

However, nothing's perfect; it can be a nuisance wearing my pump 24 hours a day. It's landed over the other side of the room after I've been spun on a night out jiving, I've woken up with it digging into my back in the middle of a deep sleep, the wires have got caught on door handles a few times and it can be difficult to hide it unobtrusively in a slinky dress. If the infusion set blocks, gets dislodged or has an air bubble and I don't receive insulin for a few hours I can go high really quickly. If I don't act on it, I will rapidly develop ketones because there is no long-acting insulin around, just rapid-acting.

It makes me feel upset that others are being denied the option of trying pump therapy. When used properly, pump therapy is the closest thing there is to normal physiology – continuous basal insulin, adjustable for different needs throughout the day, with boluses of insulin for carbo-hydrate-containing food.

Whilst insulin pumps are not for everyone, pump therapy for me did improve my HbA$_{1c}$ due to the unpredictability of my daily routine. However, much more importantly for me, it improved my quality of life.

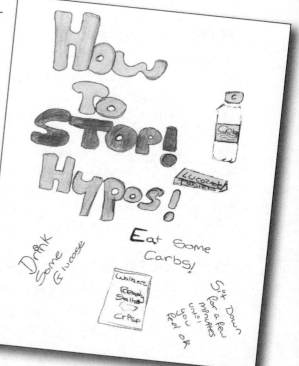

Hyperglycaemia, ketoacidosis and complications

What is hyperglycaemia?

Hyperglycaemia is a raised blood glucose, outside the normal range. It is the opposite of hypoglycaemia. In someone who doesn't have diabetes, blood glucose is tightly regulated to keep it between 4 and 7 mmol/l, as explained in more detail in Chapter 3. A value above this range is termed hyperglycaemia. After meals, blood glucose may rise but it soon goes down. Aiming for this range in someone with diabetes is not achievable all the time and should not be expected. Persistent hyperglycaemia should be avoided, but trying to avoid any raised blood glucose will result in a sense of failure and unnecessary hypoglycaemia.

What is diabetic ketoacidosis (DKA)?

Insulin is the only hormone that can lower blood glucose, and in diabetes the body does not produce insulin. Another function of insulin is to keep in balance the natural process of both protein and fat building up and breaking down. If there is not enough insulin, the balance is tipped toward protein and fat being broken down. The breakdown of fat produces ketones, which make the blood more acidic than it should be; this is ketoacidosis, also called ketosis. If the blood becomes too acidic it can be dangerous and cause reduced appetite, tummy ache, nausea, vomiting, heavy breathing and eventually unconsciousness. The ketones can be measured in the urine as well as in the blood.

How should I treat hyperglycaemia and ketoacidosis?

You will need to discuss with your diabetes team how, if and when to treat high glucose levels. Hyperglycaemia without ketones can usually be managed at home. You may not necessarily need to give extra insulin; it depends on when the blood glucose was tested and how high it is. However, any hyperglycaemia with ketones needs immediate attention to stop your child becoming ill quickly. Avoid exercise if ketones are present, or blood glucose may rise further.

What should I do if my child is unwell?

A child who has an infection may need more or less insulin than usual, depending on how the body is reacting and whether or not they can tolerate food. Even if your child is not eating, they will always need some insulin or they will rapidly develop ketones, causing diabetic ketoacidosis, and become unwell. You will need to test your child's blood glucose frequently, sometimes every hour, and make sure they are not developing ketones. Ketones can either be measured in the urine, using a dipstick, or in blood on some home blood testing machines. There is some advantage of measuring ketones in the blood as they can be picked up and acted on earlier, before they appear in the urine.

Some infections, especially those with fever, cause the release of stress hormones into the blood, and this can raise the blood glucose. If not enough insulin is given, ketones will be produced. However, in some infections, like tummy bugs, food is not well absorbed and less insulin may be needed to avoid a hypo. Even if your child is not eating, they will always need some insulin because insulin is the only hormone able to lower blood glucose.

Children who are on insulin pumps and who have a raised blood glucose need even speedier attention, because they only have fast-acting insulin, and under the effect of stress hormones they may develop ketones even faster.

Your diabetes team will be able to advise you what to do if your child is unwell. It is best to make a plan before the situation arises, as your regular diabetes team may not be available when your child falls ill. Some people call these Sick Day Rules. Sometimes, despite the plan, you may need to take your child to hospital, and you should not think of this as a failure on your part.

What are diabetic complications?

Complications are divided into those affecting blood vessels and those affecting the organs. If large blood vessels are involved, fat may be laid down in the artery wall causing it to narrow, which may lead to early heart disease, strokes, raised blood pressure or reduced blood flow to the legs.

This also happens when people smoke, whether they have diabetes or not, so smoking should be avoided if you have diabetes as it doubles the risk. Raised blood glucose also causes abnormal fat levels in the blood which can contribute to the other complications. On the other hand, healthy eating and exercise reduce the risks of heart disease and also allow for improved blood glucose control and should be encouraged.

If small blood vessels are affected, this may cause changes to the back of the eye (the retina), which can affect vision. Nerves and the kidneys may also be involved. If nerves are affected, it may be difficult to feel sensation in the feet and an injury might not be felt, which may lead to infection. Separate from complications, raised blood glucose may also affect behaviour, mood and the ability to perform some tasks.

Diabetes check-ups aim to keep an eye on diabetes control and well-being and to look out for complications so they can be prevented, reversed or treated. Normally, the Annual Review which looks for complications starts around the age of 12 in the UK, but it depends on how old your child is as well as their age at diagnosis. The Annual Review includes:

■ a blood pressure check;
■ a urine test for the kidneys;
■ an eye review by checking the eyes with a special eye photograph; and
■ a blood test.

At the same time, blood can also be checked for the activity of the thyroid and for coeliac disease, both of which can be associated with diabetes, but which are not complications of diabetes. Screening for thyroid and coeliac disease in children and young people is recommended at diagnosis and then every year for thyroid disease and at least every three years for coeliac disease.

What is the HbA$_{1c}$ and what level should be aimed for?

The HbA$_{1c}$ (short for glycoslylated haemoglobin) is a value that is used as an indirect marker of blood glucose control over a period of two to three months. Glucose in the blood sticks onto haemoglobin, a component of red blood cells. These are the cells found in blood which make the blood look red. The value of the HbA$_{1c}$ represents the proportion of red blood cells in the circulation at that time with glucose stuck to haemoglobin molecules. The HbA$_{1c}$ value reflects how blood glucose levels have been over the previous 2–3 months. However, it is just an average; if blood glucose levels frequently swing between being very high or very low, without somewhere in between, it may give you a false near-normal value.

Ideally an HbA$_{1c}$ value of 7.5% (59 mmol/mol) or less is the target, without frequent disabling hypos. Until recently HbA$_{1c}$ has been reported as a percentage, but in June 2009 it began to be reported in a different way, in mmol/mol, which is millimoles per mol. Until May 2011, both measurements will be used. This is how the two measurements compare:

HbA$_{1c}$			
%	mmol/mol	%	mmol/mol
6.0	42	8.0	64
6.5	48	9.0	75
7.0	53	10.0	86
7.5	59		

Further information can be found at www.diabetes.nhs.uk

An HbA$_{1c}$ measurement is a useful guide, although it should be interpreted in the context of each individual. Bear in mind that the figure will vary between different machines.

Who gets diabetic complications?

After a long time with diabetes, a person can expect some minor changes to blood vessels which are so small that they do not cause problems. However, complications affecting eyesight, kidney function, nerves and heart can occur over some time, which often mirror the HbA$_{1c}$. Some of these can be prevented, and if they do occur can be treated in their early stages. However, complications are not an inevitable consequence of diabetes.

There is no 'magic number' HbA$_{1c}$ at which complications never occur. However, the lower the value, the less likely it is that complications will occur at a young age and they will be less severe. Complications are not normally seen before puberty. Some people do seem to be more prone to complications than others, irrespective of HbA$_{1c}$. It is also known that a small fall in HbA$_{1c}$ will greatly reduce the risk of having complications. So that extra bit of effort is well worth it.

Case 1

The HbA$_{1c}$ and complications

Introducing Beatrice, 31, diagnosed aged 14

Three or four years ago I went to the doctor's, and when she left the room I saw in the clinic notes that she had written 'her blood sugar has never been well controlled' and that I had background retinopathy. No one had told me that I had that as a diagnosis. I thought I just had leaky vessels in my eyes. Then I had a scare with my kidneys, with protein in my urine. I had to do a 24-hour collection, but the results were OK. It's just one thing after another.

I've never reached the magic 7 [HbA$_{1c}$], but if I did I'd feel like I'd achieved something. But I'm not on any medication for my blood pressure and my cholesterol is perfect.

I've never had DKA [diabetic ketoacidosis] because I check my sugars and if I'm high I correct it straight away. Not a day's gone by when I haven't checked my blood sugar twice a day. I consider myself relatively well-controlled when there are people out there with HbA$_{1c}$s in the teens.

My ultimate fear is getting kidney failure and blindness. It doesn't matter how well-controlled you can get your blood sugar, you can still get complications. If I knew that if I had a certain HbA$_{1c}$ I wouldn't get complications, I would act on it. But you get up and do your blood. It may be 5, 6 or 7. Later you might be high and have to act on it. Then you go through the rest of the day. You have to do the same thing tomorrow and the next day. The day after that you have to do it all again. It's always one step ahead of you, you are always having to work towards it.

The hardest thing is trying to act accordingly now – it's difficult to carry out an action that may have its results in 30 years' time.

When I went through my kidney scare I said 'I'm never eating chocolate again!' But by the end of the day I'd crave chocolate and buy a Twix. So now I eat a small Penguin bar every day.

They [the doctors] don't know what it's like to try and control it. You're just another set of figures. They don't know how hard it is. You wake up each day and have to do the same thing all over again.

Case 1 *continued*

I used to see a doctor and didn't like him at all. It was all about figures rather than looking at your whole lifestyle and how diabetes could fit in with your life, and not the other way around. Now I see my GP. He's kind and compassionate.

I think they [the doctors] do know if you try and look after yourself or if you don't give a shit. Sometimes I'd just like some acknowledgement of how hard I try.

Discussion

Having hyperglycaemia – raised blood glucose levels – at times is an inevitable part of living with diabetes, just as it is to have low blood glucose levels – hypoglycaemia. Although it often does not feel like it, there will always be a reason for the blood glucose level, although unpicking the reason can be tricky.

You and your child will have been told what a 'normal' blood glucose level is and what blood glucose level to aim for. When those goals are not met, your child may feel like they are a 'bad diabetic', a failure. Trying as hard as you can and still getting it wrong can make you and your child feel frustrated, sad and angry; you feel as though you have done something wrong.

Beatrice in Case 1 feels that she has never achieved her goal of a 'perfect' HbA_{1c}, the 'magic 7'. It feels unreachable to her. It also feels a bit pointless, since it does not guarantee her freedom from complications. She also feels that because she has not reached her target she is judged negatively by her diabetes team, despite working hard at her diabetes, day in, day out. This only further increases her anxiety about complications. She seems to act on any raised glucose levels and there is an overriding feeling that her diabetes is always one step ahead of her.

Beatrice found out about her diabetic complications in a shocking way; she now has no empathy with her diabetes team. She feels they do not acknowledge her efforts, so she has gone elsewhere, to her GP. When your child finds out even about the possibility they could have complications, let alone getting them, it is a real blow. It is like having a diagnosis for the first time. A child as young as 7 may in this way become aware of their own mortality. This is an uncommon experience for a child, and is bound to change a young person's experience of the world as they grow up.

Case 2

The conflict of blood glucose control and complications

Introducing Jason, 27, diagnosed aged 7

In some ways when I was growing up I ignored the focus on control as I thought, because I could do everything, that I was normal, then all these things wouldn't happen to me.

My biggest fear is going blind and having my legs chopped off – I'd shoot myself. I'd never had a proper eye review. Recently I had a scan after I asked to be referred from my GP to the hospital. I was told that I had spots at the back of my eyes but they are reversible. I freaked out, but then again I wasn't that surprised after having diabetes for 20 years.

Trying to manage the diabetes really well and do a job at the same time is difficult. If other things are on, they take priority. It [diabetes control] should be at the forefront of my mind. I think that if I had a simple life with less stress... But then I could wrap myself up in cotton wool, but what kind of life is that? Given the choice I'd prefer an interesting life that's a bit shorter. Diabetes is something that might end my life, but then again there are so many other things that might too.

Discussion

Jason, and Beatrice in the previous case, are now adults and have made the decision to have less tight blood glucose control and what they see as a more fulfilled life. They do not feel that this is compatible with achieving tight blood glucose control, even though their ultimate fear is of complications.

Since one of the easiest ways to achieve diabetes control is through routine, they are likely making the decision to have less routine and a more flexible life. The conflict between ignoring the diabetes and 'doing whatever you like' is one that many young people and adults with diabetes go through. Clearly, a balance must be struck because long-term poor control brings complications. And the complications, if they continue, may cause a burden and might interrupt this flexibility too. Hyperglycaemia itself can cause feelings of poor energy and not feeling 100% well, which could also impact on daily life. On the other side, concentrating solely on blood glucose control to the detriment of enjoying life is seen by some as pointless. After all, what is the point of having no complications if you are miserable or bored?

Both ends of the spectrum are extreme examples; a balance between them must be found. So long as your child is young enough to be under your control, you may struggle with this conflict too. It may be easier for you when you have complete control of your child, but as they grow up and start becoming independent, you lose control and may feel helpless to prevent them from getting complications.

Jason and Beatrice's choice is in part determined by the uncertainty and unpredictability of complications. Beatrice would like to be guaranteed that if she works hard to achieve a blood glucose number she will avoid complications. Since there is no such guarantee, she makes the decision to tilt the balance in favour of less rigidity in her life at the risk of running higher blood glucose levels.

Jason's experience is slightly different. He wants to be 'normal', which in his mind is being able to do anything that someone without diabetes can do. For him this was a more important focus when growing up, rather than a specific blood glucose number. He voices a recurring theme in this book, of feeling and being different but not wanting to be seen as different.

Case 3

Behaviour changes with high blood glucose levels

Introducing Kiet, 16, diagnosed aged 15

I feel proper angry when I'm high and my adrenaline's rushing. I do stupid stuff. I don't know what I'm doing. Anyone who talks to me, I confront them. I run around and terrorise the other children in school, throwing conkers and slide-tackling them. When I did that my blood sugar on the machine said 'HI'. I got excluded for five days.

Discussion

Kiet is aware of how his high glucose levels affect his behaviour and impact on his life at school. As a parent you will want to protect your child from harm, but it is frustrating when they don't do what you want them to do. Kiet is a teenager and cannot foresee the risk of his raised blood glucose levels more than in the short term. He denies to himself the impact that hyperglycaemia has so much that he refuses to prevent it by taking his injections.

Although good glucose control does not necessarily guarantee freedom from complications, it does make them much less likely to happen, and if they do, they will be less severe.

Q **What does it feel like to have a high blood sugar?**

A How someone feels with a raised blood glucose level will depend on them individually as a person. It will also depend on how long they have had the high glucose level and whether ketones are present.

Your child may not feel any different if the high glucose level is, for example, just after a meal and they have had some insulin. If you check the blood glucose two hours later, it may be nearer normal. However, if the glucose has been high for some time, causing the child to pass urine frequently, they may also start to feel thirsty and dehydrated with a headache. If there is not enough insulin in the body, the fat stores will start to produce ketones which can cause tummy ache, nausea and vomiting. Ketones also reduce appetite, so they might not be at all hungry. It would be a good idea to ask yourself whether this is in keeping with your child's normal behaviour.

How someone feels will depend on their normal blood glucose level. For example, if your child's blood glucose is normally around 12 mmol/l, then having a blood glucose of 15 mmol/l may not feel particularly different. However, if they have a blood glucose that is normally around 6 mmol/l they may really notice the change. Some people have a blood glucose of 15 or more all the time, and feel perfectly all right: the body seems to adapt. They often feel 'grotty' if their sugar falls to 7 mmol/l.

continued

Compare hyperglycaemia to a mild hypo, which tends to be immediate; if you are hypo you can't carry on, but if you eat something then you're back to normal. For many people, if you're high the feeling tends to last longer, probably because it creeps up on you more slowly, and you can carry on even if you are a bit sluggish.

Remember that blood test results are a snapshot of the glucose level at just one moment in time; a reading of 18 mmol/l may be on the way down if taken just after a meal with an injection, or on the way up if just before supper if on a twice-a-day regimen.

With my old insulin regime I was always high before my evening meal. I wouldn't feel like eating. I kept having this cycle when I wouldn't eat dinner and then about an hour later after I'd done my injection I'd be really hungry. Mum found it a bit frustrating.

(Jason, 27)

What does hyperglycaemia feel like?

Here is a selection of responses from those with diabetes about what being hyperglycaemic feels like to them.

A bit tired, same as when I'm low.

(Margaret, 12)

Even worse than a hypo, I get a bad belly ache and headaches.

(Janina, 13)

Thirsty and really tired.

(Beatrice, 31)

Lethargic, tired and lazy. It's not good for my school work.

(Luke, 17)

I get a burning feeling in my chest and feel really hot and so, so tired.

(Lizzie, 27)

Thirsty. I have to go to the toilet a lot.

(Jeffrey, 9)

I hate it, it's so uncomfortable. I get this disgusting taste in my mouth. I get really grouchy, lethargic, not wanting to speak to people, lackadaisical, my muscles ache, I don't feel hungry and I can't eat anything. Sometimes I get confused with being high or low, the symptoms can be similar.

(Jason, 27)

A really bad beer hangover with a headache, really really depressed and a lack of energy... awful, no appetite, sick, constantly thirsty.

(Martina, 28)

I get absolutely exhausted. Even climbing the stairs is too much. It's a horrible, horrible feeling.

(Nigel, 37)

I can run 22 [mmol/l] and not notice it or I can get pains in my legs and be lethargic.

(George, 35)

My head gets muggy, I can't focus and I get moody at work. It's a massive relief when I do my injection knowing that in 20 minutes from now I'll start to feel better.

(Lucia, 37)

I feel tired, as if I've run a long distance and I'm numb all over my body. It lasts as long as my blood's high. The worst is if I'm high all night and wake up with a high blood. But if I'm high in the day I give some insulin and start feeling better as my blood starts to come down.

(Flin, 23)

Q **When is the right time to talk to my child about complications?**

A Most children are unaware of their mortality. Yet on asking young people with diabetes about what they are most worried about related to their diabetes, the fear of hypos and complications comes up time and again. Children as young as 12 years old speak about their fear of dying (see Chapter 11: The best and worst of times).

As a parent you might sometimes get frustrated, and be tempted to use the risk of complications as a scare tactic to try to get your child to look after their diabetes better. When your child was diagnosed you may have grieved the loss of your 'healthy' child. Knowing that complications are out there and may happen may make you feel helpless, anxious and angry. You will want to do everything in your power to prevent the complications and protect your child from harm. Every high glucose reading may feel like a step closer to complications. This is a bit melodramatic and is dealt with in a later question. However, it may be a reason, when you are frustrated and worried, to warn your child about the future if they do not take better care.

It is difficult to know when to talk about complications. If you say nothing, they may find out anyway and it can be a big shock. Finding out from others can be frightening; worse, the information might be incorrect, based on perceptions of diabetes over the past 50 years, when complications were more common and more severe and diabetes treatment was less sophisticated. Using scare tactics never works, and can have the opposite effect: making your child frightened or stressed, and even rebellious. If your child feels that complications are inevitable, then there is little point in trying.

You will need to introduce the idea early that raised blood glucose levels are not good for the body and try to let your child see that when their blood glucose levels are well-controlled they feel better and can do more. Perhaps demonstrate they can concentrate better at school, have a better night's sleep or run faster on the football pitch.

Mum says if I eat too much chocolate I'll die.

(Darren, 12)

I was first told about complications when I was 7. 'You might go blind if you don't treat it right'. Then when I was 10 or 11 my paediatric nurse told me I should practice my injection in the dark in case I go blind. It made me feel scared. I put it at the back of my mind.

(Jason, 27)

If someone said you could have one or the other [diabetes or blindness] to take away, I'd say the diabetes every time. Blindness is a problem because of the outside world but diabetes is debilitating because it affects you internally and in your body.

(Martina, 28)

Mum says if you don't look after your diabetes your feet are going to drop off and you'll go blind. If my feet hurt or ache I'm scared - I think they're going to fall off. That's why I want to be healthier 'cos I don't want to go blind.

(Summer, 13)

Q Jack checks his blood sugars six times a day. What's the point in checking them so often when they are high most of the time?

A Checking blood glucose levels does not necessarily ensure good blood glucose control unless they are looked at, thought about and acted upon. Some people check the blood glucose levels but don't record them; this seems a bit pointless, but is understandable when you consider the fact that it must be done day in, day out. These days we have blood glucose meters that record results, with the

A *continued*

dates and times, and these can be downloaded onto computers at home or in the hospital outpatient clinic.

I wonder why Jack checks his blood six times a day and whether he acts on the results, or whether you do. Is he worried about being low or high? Perhaps he is not yet old enough to work out what he needs to do to improve his glucose readings. You will need to help him; and you will need the help of your diabetes team. They may be able to look at the blood glucose results and see a pattern emerging which may be difficult for you to see, in close range and living with Jack's diabetes every day.

If my blood sugars are constantly high or low I panic in case I go into a coma.

(Margaret, 12)

Q I can see that Anne (13) doesn't like being high and worries about complications in the future. So why doesn't she control her blood sugars better?

A Knowing what you need to do is one thing; actually doing them is something else entirely. The daily grind of trying to keep stable blood glucose levels can seem like hard work, especially as it's endless. Like Beatrice in Case 1, many young people with diabetes would like encouragement and their efforts acknowledged. Often this is self-reinforcing: if you feel better you are motivated to do more and make more effort.

Perhaps Anne has other fears, such as the fear of having hypos. She may need more support or positive encouragement. Sharing experiences with others in the same situation can help reduce the stress and anxiety, both for Anne and yourself. Relieving this stress by sharing experiences may allow a more open discussion between you about the real problems.

Also, with everything else that is going on in living life – school

continued on next page

continued

work, friends, sleepovers, being part of a family – it is not surprising that diabetes, which lasts forever, takes the back burner from something that needs more pressing attention, like passing a French spelling test or finding a birthday present for Dad.

I make excuses to myself. Like today I tell myself I've been busy. I'd like to get good end results without having to do all the tests. I can't contemplate complications. They said I had to keep it under control but most of the time I can't be bothered.

(Luke, 17)

I worry about hypos in case I can't treat it in time and go unconscious or it happens when I am at work – it'd be embarrassing or I might make a weird decision. At the same time I am petrified of getting complications. But the complications seem so far away and the fear of hypos is every day.

(Susie, 24)

If I was a good boy and led a restricted life I might not have complications. But I wasn't prepared to do it. I wanted to live a normal life – to live my life normally like anyone else.

(George, 35, who has retinopathy in his right eye)

I've had diabetes for 34 years and have no complications. The secret is to get a life and get a grip. I can live with diabetes and have conquered it. It's all about acceptance.

(Nigel, 37)

Q Am I right to panic every time Joe gets a high blood glucose reading?

A This is an easy thing to do, especially at the beginning when your child has just been diagnosed. I expect you will have been told what a normal blood glucose is and what to aim for, and why. When there is a reading outside that range it may seem like you have failed, and some parents even imagine the complications happening in front of their eyes with each raised blood glucose reading.

Let's put things into perspective. The problems which give rise to complications are cumulative. The best thing you can do is to try to understand why the blood glucose is high and anticipate whether any changes need be made for next time, rather than panicking and overreacting to it. For example, maybe you needed to give a bit more insulin when he was eating a larger quantity of carbohydrate, or maybe he didn't need such a large snack before exercise. If you are not used to doing this, or are not yet confident at doing this alone or with Joe, your diabetes team will help.

You don't need to panic; there is time for you to become skilled at understanding diabetes and working out the reason for Joe's blood glucose levels and when things need to change. You don't need to be an expert straight away and you can still keep him safe while you all learn about diabetes together. The process of paying attention and thinking and talking things through will bring benefits in the long run, so you and your child can be in charge of the diabetes; you will be able to anticipate changes in insulin and/or food in response to different situations, and Joe will be able to live an independent life.

Here is a useful checklist of questions to ask when confronted by a raised blood glucose level.

■ Is the blood glucose level potentially dangerously high (greater than 17 mmol/l, or 14 mmol/l on an insulin pump)? If so, check for ketones in the blood or urine. If there are ketones, seek medical advice.

■ Did they take their insulin? If so, was it the right type, in the right amount, and could it have been injected into a site that doesn't absorb insulin well, like a fatty lump?

continued on next page

continued

- How soon after eating was the blood glucose reading taken? If it was within a couple of hours and the insulin was given, wait. As a rule try not to test within two hours of eating as it is likely to be above the normal range and then may well be normal in a couple of hours.
- Reacting to a raised blood glucose level in this situation by giving extra insulin too early may result in a hypo.
- When was their last hypo? Could the effect you're seeing be because of rebound? (See Chapter 2: Hypoglycaemia.)
- Could they be ill, for example with an infection?

I feel guilty when I'm high.

(Flin, 23)

Q **We go to clinic and the doctors tells Simon that he needs to control his blood sugars better but he won't listen. He is 17 and I am scared of what the future holds. How can I get through to him?**

A Young people may have had negative experiences with healthcare professionals when they were diagnosed. They may feel that their diabetes team do not really understand about their diabetes or what it feels like, and just seem to be there to tell them off. Many young people think, 'What do they know about my diabetes? I know more about it than them!' In many ways they are right. No one really knows except for that person with diabetes: what it feels like, what they ate, where they injected, if they have stress hormones whizzing around their body. Going to clinic can seem like the time when they are always told they must do better, when there is always something that could be improved upon. It is the time when complications are looked for; if there are none, the team will continue to look for them until they arrive, which may be never. All the things you must do,

continued

and not do, are rolled out again. There is little acknowledgement of the hard work you do every day with diabetes, which is added to the list of other demands: do your homework, tidy your room, eat this or don't eat that, at that time of day.

Ideally, you and your child will become the experts. The doctors, nurses and dietitians will guide and advise, but can only do so with your help. As a team you are a powerful combination – with you and your child's personal knowledge and experience, coupled with your diabetes team's general and collective experience of dealing with many other children and young people in a similar situation. However, neither work as well alone as they can do together, as long as both sides are listening to each other.

Children are harsh judges. One negative event – a comment or even a look – can turn a child off their diabetes team forever, losing the child's trust. That might be a good reason, to a child, why not to follow their rules. Often it is one thing that a child or adult with diabetes remembers from a clinic appointment – perhaps it is the way a doctor listened or asked a question, even one unrelated to their diabetes.

However, if you and your child can be an equal partnership with your diabetes team you will be a powerful combination and one in which diabetes plays second fiddle to leading a fulfilling life.

To have diabetes you have to go to hospital, you take your level and see how it's been every three months. It's very hard having diabetes. You have to deal with a lot of things. As you get older you have to take a lot of responsibility. When you go to clinic you have to listen to what they say.

(Jeffrey, 9)

You go for your check-ups and say 'Oh yes' and then you go home and do your own thing. There's no point in arguing with them.

(Mike, 27)

Every clinic they would talk about complications. I thought they were obsessed with complications as if they were waiting for them to happen. If I didn't have any, it was like, 'Not yet, oh well, wait till next time'. It was as if they were waiting to chop your legs off. You need to be aware but you assume it's not something that'd happen today or tomorrow. Now I go to the adult clinic and they seem to know what they're talking about, or perhaps I am more open to their advice as I am older. I am willing to discuss things now and don't necessarily think I know more than they do.

(Jason, 27)

What you can do

- **Try and be positive**. Reward your child for good behaviour, rather than concentrating on blood glucose levels.
- **Acknowledge that you appreciate the daily grind and hard work.** After all, you probably share in it as well.
- **Try and be proactive rather than reactive.** You will need to react when there are ketones present and very high blood glucose levels. However, at other times you might be better off recording the level and then taking an overview to see if a trend emerges.
- **Do not use scare tactics** to get your child to follow diabetes advice – it never helps and often does more harm than good. The cases and quotes in this chapter demonstrate that young children have memories about specific things they were told and these may stick with them, consciously or subconsciously, all their lives.
- **Try and help your child to achieve as near normal blood glucose levels as possible.** This will make them feel better, affect their behaviour and lower their risk of long-term complications.
- **Ask your diabetes team about the Sick Day Rules.** These tell you what to do if your child is unwell, and if he or she is unwell and not eating. You will feel less scared when you have a plan in place. If the plan is not effective, you may need to go to hospital. This sometimes just happens and is not a failure on your part.

Here is an example of how you might introduce the idea of complications. This will need to be changed according to the age of your child and what they already know.

> ❝ If your blood glucose is raised a lot of the time, after many years this may affect some parts of your body. To stop that from happening, the doctors check that you are OK once a year. If there is a problem they will spot it, and it will be treated. Or it may be a reminder to tell us to keep the blood sugars down a bit. In the meantime, with the doctors, nurses and dietitians, we will help to keep your blood sugar levels down as much as possible. Having a one-off high isn't a big deal and is no one's fault. We can think about why it has happened to try to stop it happening again. Also, if the high blood sugar makes you feel tired it's not a very nice feeling. But it is all practice. You are doing brilliantly at your injections/blood tests and even if your blood tests are high, it is not your fault as you did not ask to have diabetes. ❞

I'd have liked them to be more positive and concentrate more on managing the diabetes with the focus on better control.

(Jason, 27)

Don't paint the worst case scenario. It's like saying that if I have asthma, my lungs might collapse. If you don't abuse your diabetes it won't lead to complications. Complications don't worry me.

(Nigel, 37)

Rachel's view

I don't like feeling high, it makes me feel slow. I also don't like feeling low. I like to be just right. It's tempting to run a bit high to avoid hypos in certain situations but with practice I can get my bloods spot on – but not all of the time. The difference I feel when my bloods are steadily normal compared to running high is enormous. I have this huge amount of energy that is zapped away when they go up. My bloods still go high but I know how to correct them. I've had some blips with my bloods going high for longer periods, when life has been stressful and my diabetes has not been my priority. I have to retame them then. You can try to ignore diabetes for a bit but not for too long. I've learnt it's better to accept it's there and work with it, allow it to be your friend so the two of you don't argue too much.

I feel furious when I hear young children talking about how they have been scared by talk of complications. They are so frightened and that doesn't improve their blood glucose levels, it often makes them worse.

Complications do worry me but the fear is probably worse than the reality. Every year at my Annual Review I worry that I'll be told that this is the year that I have started to get complications. I sit in the waiting room trying not to worry. When I get my eyes checked, I make my eye doctor check again for me. He laughs when I ask him, 'Are you sure there's not even a dot, would you like to look again?' I did get a dot once when I had glandular fever and had fevers for a few months. My bloods were difficult to control and my HbA_{1c} shot up. I got a dot then but it went away when my bloods normalised and has stayed away.

When I go for my Annual Review, I like to see the results written down so I can digest them. When I leave with (touch wood) no complications, I walk away lighter in step, with the worry removed for another year. If I do get complications, it would be a really big deal. I would feel as though I had failed and that it was my fault. I would be devastated. It would be as though the diabetes had won.

School

How much diabetes care and support should I expect from school?

There are no standardised care policies for managing diabetes in UK schools. How much care and support children need will depend on their insulin regimen, knowledge, diabetes stability, age and length of diagnosis. Many schools are fantastic at helping young people adjust to life with diabetes. However, others are less open to support and this can cause distress, affect diabetes control and even cause parents to leave work in order to take on health responsibilities in school.

Individual schools may have a policy and this will vary according to the philosophy of the school, which may be in part to do with knowledge and previous experience. Your paediatric diabetes nurse will need to engage well with the school in order to meet the health needs of your child.

There are various legal standards that relate to children with diabetes worth knowing about: a few are explained below. A fuller explanation can be found in a Diabetes UK document *Making all children matter: Support for children with diabetes in schools*, which can be downloaded from the Diabetes UK website.

Disability Discrimination Act (DDA) 1995

Most adults and children with diabetes do not see themselves as disabled. However, diabetes is included under this Act because 'without adequate treatment it will cause significant and long-term adverse effects on the ability to carry out normal day-to-day activities'. This means that if you have diabetes you are protected from discrimination under the DDA.

Special Educational Needs and Disability Act 2001

This is intended to prohibit discrimination in school against children who are disabled, and covers children with diabetes. Schools are not required to provide extra services, but they also cannot discriminate against someone either by treating them less favourably or by not taking reasonable steps to make sure that pupils are not at a disadvantage. I consider that a child running high blood glucose levels is at a disadvantage. Not checking blood glucose levels in order to act to reduce them to improve that child's health and learning potential discriminates against that child. However, Local Education Authorities (LEAs) have 'a duty not to treat disabled pupils less favourably, without justification, for a reason which relates to their disability', which includes making 'reasonable adjustments'.

Schools can apply for funding via an LEA, for example to train staff in supervision of insulin administration, choosing correct snacks, supervising or performing blood glucose tests. Enforcement is via a tribunal. However, Local Authorities may say that care should be provided by school and school may say they do not have the resources to do so, which is an unsatisfactory situation. Some schools, such as foundation schools and voluntary aided schools, do not necessarily have to answer to an LEA, but to the governing body, which may make the application process more complicated.

The Children Act 1989 and 2004

The 1989 Act gives local authorities responsibility to 'safeguard and promote the welfare of children within their area who are in need...by providing a range and level of services appropriate to those children's needs'.

The Children Act 2004 provided the legal foundation for development of the government document *Every Child Matters; Change for Children*. One key area of this document relevant to children with diabetes in school is for 'a duty on Local Authorities to make arrangements to promote co-operation between agencies and other appropriate bodies to...improve children's well-being'.

Department for Education and Skills

In 2005, guidelines were produced on the administration of medicines in schools (*Managing Medicines in Schools and Early Years Settings*). The relevant sections related to diabetes care are listed below, but they are contradictory. It may be worth pointing out to the people concerned at school that extremes of blood sugar, i.e. hypoglycaemia and hyper-glycaemia *are emergencies*.

- Para 16: There is no legal duty that requires school or other educational setting staff to administer medicines.

- Para 87: All staff should be aware of the likelihood of an emergency arising and what action to take if one occurs.

- Para 89: Teachers' conditions of employment do not include giving or supervising a pupil taking medicines. Schools should ensure that they have sufficient members of support staff who are employed and appropriately trained to manage medicines as part of their duties.

- Para 90: Any member of staff who agrees to accept responsibility for administering prescribed medicines to a child should have appropriate training and guidance.

- Para 111: Children need to have immediate access to their medicines when required. The school or setting may want to make special access arrangements for an emergency.

Using this information

Ideally you, your diabetes team and school will work well together. However, if difficulties arise it is good to know that your child is covered by legislation, and this information is a good starting point for finding help. It is best not to resort to the law, as it can harm your relationship with the school. However, you should not give up on your aim to keep your child safe at school and in good health. At the end of this chapter is a suggested framework for approaching schools for the first time.

Does diabetes affect a child's ability to learn and reach their full potential?

Both low and high blood glucose can affect a child's learning and their ability to access the curriculum. In the immediate term, hypoglycaemia needs treatment because if it is not treated a child may become unconscious. If the blood glucose is raised this may affect a child's ability to learn and perform tasks. In the longer term, the effects of hyperglycaemia may cause diabetic complications such as heart disease, damage to eyes, kidneys and nerves. Complications will probably not happen during a child's time at school, but knowing what the blood glucose level is in school will allow you and the diabetes team to make changes to a child's insulin dose and dietary advice to increase a child's learning ability and reduce the occurrence of hypoglycaemia, hyperglycaemia and longer-term diabetic complications.

School is a great opportunity to bring stability and routine into a life with diabetes – breaks and lunch are at the same time every day and exercise can usually be anticipated through the timetable.

What do I need to consider when my child goes to school?

There are lots of issues to think about, none of which need to be a major problem.

When should a child's blood glucose be tested?

Your child should have the facility to have a blood glucose test in the following situations:

- If they don't feel right: to confirm what their blood glucose level is. It should not be assumed a child is hypo if they 'feel funny' because these feelings can be confused with having a high blood glucose level, and the treatments are different.
- Before lunch and before PE. This is necessary in order to optimise blood glucose control to avoid hypoglycaemia and hyperglycaemia.

Where should blood testing occur?

Blood glucose testing should ideally occur at your child's desk because if their blood glucose level is low, walking to another room to test may make them even lower. If this is not possible in school, they should be accompanied by an adult (not a child) to a designated place where a blood glucose test can be performed.

What happens once the blood test has been performed?

A Health Care Plan should be in place to decide what action (if any) is needed to act on hypoglycaemia or hyperglycaemia.

Hypoglycaemia (low blood glucose levels)

Treatment should be readily available to your child in case of hypo-glycaemia. This could be held by your child or a teacher, but must be readily available once hypoglycaemia is confirmed by blood glucose testing.

Hyperglycaemia (raised blood glucose levels)

If your child needs to go to the toilet during class they should be allowed to do so because raised blood glucose levels will cause an increased need to pass urine. Once your child has passed urine they should perform a blood glucose test to confirm if the blood glucose is raised in order to make any necessary adjustments.

Your child's insulin regimen will dictate how rigid they will need to be about timings of snacks and any need to eat during class. Support in choosing appropriate snacks may also be needed.

Injections

If your child needs a lunchtime injection, this should occur at a suitable place that should interfere as little as possible with school life. This may be at the dinner table, just before or just after eating, depending on the Health Care Plan, or they may find themselves at the back of the dinner queue having a hypo. You also need to think about the exercise your child takes, in terms of insulin and/or food adjustments.

Exams

Exam time needs special consideration; having a hypo or a high blood glucose during an exam can affect a child's performance. For the actual exam, your child will need to be equipped with snacks and a blood testing kit. I have never heard of anyone not being allowed these in an exam. Extra time may be needed during an exam, especially if they have a hypo and need time to recover, although this is rarely thought about. High blood glucose in an exam may adversely affect a child's ability to perform and should be noted. Stress hormones can cause blood glucose levels to run high, especially with nerves just before an exam, although this is sometimes only transient. Also, if your child is usually active, sitting in an exam hall for a whole morning or afternoon can cause blood glucose to run high. You can prepare for these eventualities by thinking ahead, knowing your child and getting help from your diabetes team and support from school.

School trips

A good school will make reasonable adjustments to make sure your child is not left out. Many parents with younger children go on the trip with them, especially if it's only a day trip. Sometimes, unfortunately, schools may try to pressure you not to send your child on a school trip, or say they cannot go. No school is allowed to discriminate against a child with diabetes under the DDA.

Emotional well-being

Children and young people with diabetes do not like to feel different from their peers just because they have diabetes and should not be encouraged to behave differently. Minimising this will encourage a young person to comply with diabetes treatment in the short and longer term. For example, some children may deliberately miss injections to avoid their friends knowing they have diabetes.

Each individual child will have an opinion on how they would like to be treated in school. Some like a special pass which means they can leave class a bit early for a lunchtime injection without being singled out whereas others are happy to have an injection at the dinner table. Make sure you and your child are brought into the discussion regarding the above situations in order to comply with management and feel part of the decision-making process.

Young people with diabetes can go on to achieve just as much as their peers without diabetes, but this will only be possible with good blood glucose control.

> I used to go into exams loaded up with sweets. I would run high so I didn't go hypo in the middle of an exam.
>
> *(Beatrice, 31)*

> I had a hypo in an exam and had to stop for ten minutes. I didn't say anything as I didn't like to think of my diabetes as a hindrance.
>
> *(Flin, 23)*

Case 1

Diabetes in school

Introducing Mike, 27, diagnosed aged 11

I was diagnosed at the beginning of my secondary school, two weeks into the beginning of term. I was known as the 'ill-looking child'. When I went back to school all the friendship groups had already formed. People were going out at weekends, but I wasn't invited. I never really caught up. I still feel pissed off about it.

If I couldn't or didn't want to do something, teachers would suggest it was because of my diabetes. I just went along with it. In PE, I could avoid doing some of the activities. I remember everyone having to do a full length in the hall of forward rolls, but I only had to do one. I was happy at the time because I didn't like doing forward rolls. Sometimes I would get told off if I ate in class and the teachers forgot I was diabetic, but my friends would stick up for me.

There had been another boy in the school with diabetes, two years older than me. When my teacher found out I was diabetic he said, 'You're not like him, he was a bad diabetic'. I realised that he didn't know anything about diabetes.

Discussion

School is a major part of a child's life and so is having diabetes: they need to work well together. Children can have a variable response to their diabetes in school: one day Mike could use his diabetes as an excuse to opt out of PE, another day he was told off for eating in class. This reflects different teachers' understanding and knowledge.

Even in a school that has had a child with diabetes before, statistically there will probably only be one child or at most two at any one time with diabetes. Just like Mike's teacher, many people without diabetes think that how many hypos or injections someone with diabetes has reflects how badly affected they are. Mike's teacher thought that the other boy had diabetes more severely because he had more hypos or he had to inject at lunchtime, whereas at the time Mike did not. It only goes to show what a lack of understanding there is about diabetes and will also explain why Mike received such a varying response to his diabetes.

Case 2

Injecting in school and dealing with questions

Introducing Margaret, 12, diagnosed aged 2

It was only in Year 6 [10–11 year olds] that I had to inject in school. I had to run down to the Medical Room to do my injection. Now I carry a Red Pass and leave class a bit early. When I first did that they asked 'Where'd you go?!' I told them and now they don't ask me any more.

Some people ask me loads of questions, like 'What is diabetes?' 'What is a hypo?' 'What is insulin?' Sometimes they ask me the same question every time and go on and on when I'm trying to think.

Once in Year 5 or 6 someone said 'I know why Margaret's got diabetes – it's 'cos her Mum stabbed her when she was little'. It went round all the school and someone told me. I didn't take any notice. I said [to her], 'I didn't get stabbed'. I told her about diabetes. At the end of the day we're all human beings.

Discussion

Margaret was diagnosed at a younger age than Mike and doesn't remember much about life before diabetes. She experienced name-calling but because she understands about diabetes well she was able to explain all about it. Her school has allowed her to carry a pass to allow her to be excused from class to do a lunchtime blood test and injection without explaining herself every day, avoiding making a bigger deal out of it than it is.

Case 3

Diabetes in school

Introducing Daniel, 17, diagnosed aged 12

When I was at secondary school I found it hard to fit in. Before lunch I had to go downstairs to the Medical Room to do my injection so I ended up eating lunch on my own. I didn't like it at all. Then the diabetes specialist nurse sorted me on three injections a day, one in the morning, one at supper and one at bed, so it sorted it out. I had

Case 3 *continued*

friends to sit with at lunch. But it didn't help me health-wise as my blood sugars ran high by the evening, but if I gave more insulin in the morning I'd be hypo at lunchtime.

Once I had an accident in school. I was sitting in French class and my blood sugar was really high. I needed to go to the toilet. I asked the teacher and he asked if I could hold it but it started to get really bad. The teacher said 'No'. Then it happened. I walked out. People said something about me having a weak bladder.

If they see me having a hypo and eating sweets they'll come over and ask 'Why you doing that?' At certain times I don't want to reveal my whole life. They might know I'm diabetic but they've never seen the consequences.

I think teachers need to be better educated about diabetes during their studies or on a special teacher-training day.

Discussion

While some people are given the option to use their diabetes as an excuse, Daniel experienced the other extreme; he was not listened to at school and his diabetes was not properly considered. His teacher may have forgotten he had diabetes – Daniel has done a good job of trying to fit in and be 'normal'. This is a hard message for teachers – treat children with diabetes normally and don't give them excuses, but at the same time be considerate and remember they have diabetes and may need attention or to leave class when they would otherwise not be allowed to. Unfortunately, Daniel probably had a high blood glucose level that day and filled up his bladder quickly; he really did need to go to the toilet.

Daniel's diabetes nurse had changed his insulin regimen. On the one hand this fitted in with Daniel's needs and wants; he didn't have to inject at lunchtime or pay much attention to his diabetes around his friends during the school day. On the other hand, this insulin regimen wasn't ideal for him because the morning dose made the day less flexible; Daniel tried to juggle being too low at lunchtime with being high in the afternoon and early evening. A four-times-a-day insulin regimen, with a long-acting injection in the evening and rapid-acting injections at mealtimes, would suit Daniel's blood glucose levels better. If he could be persuaded to try it he might feel much better, which may be the motivation for doing his lunchtime injection. However, if he feels so strongly that he doesn't want others to see his injection or to be different, he may choose to miss his lunchtime injection and run high all afternoon causing the same difficulties.

Q Kelly is changing to secondary school soon and does her own injections. She doesn't want anyone in her new school to know she has diabetes. I don't feel this is safe. Should I follow her wishes or put my foot down?

A Many children do not want to tell their friends that they have diabetes and so they go to lengths to hide it. Unless something is said or something happens, like a hypo, no one will be any the wiser. Diabetes is one of many 'hidden disabilities'. On the outside your child is no different, but on the inside their diabetes does make them different, which may make them feel differently about their body and their identity.

If it's handled well, and the decision comes from your child, telling people at school doesn't have to cause great anxiety. Other children may forget about it completely once the initial information is given.

Your child may have had a previous uncomfortable experience related to their diabetes. Perhaps they have been called names or teased over food. They may hate the continual questions from curious classmates, however well-meaning they may be, and start feeling as though their diabetes defines them. They may already be experiencing 'diabetic burnout' – the annoyance of having to think and talk about diabetes all the time. If telling all is going to change how your child is treated, it is not surprising that they want to keep it a secret. However, it is likely to come out eventually, for example if they have a hypo in school.

Often when children find out about a classmate's diabetes, the child in question has great novelty value. But if diabetes is not explained to them properly, inaccuracies spread like Chinese whis-

A continued

pers and can cause distress. People get wrong ideas from knowing another person with diabetes, perhaps an elderly relative with Type 2 diabetes. Maybe a classmate hears the word 'diabetes' and asks a parent about it, to be told, for example, that having diabetes means that you're not allowed to eat sweets.

Type 2 diabetes can occur, less frequently, in children. Whereas Type 1 diabetes is caused by an almost complete deficiency of insulin, in Type 2 the person does produce some insulin but it cannot be used properly in the body. The end result is similar: hyper-glycaemia, but the treatment is different. Type 2 is treated by dietary modification and tablets, as well as insulin sometimes too. Also, if someone with Type 1 misses taking their insulin, they can become ill quite quickly, but in Type 2 diabetes not complying with diet or missing a tablet will not be so harmful in the short term.

A child with diabetes has to juggle the demands of diabetes, correcting other people's attitudes, making friends and coping with the demands of school. It says a lot for children with diabetes that many go through school without much thought or too much fuss about their diabetes.

It would be worth asking Kelly why she doesn't want to tell school. It might just be that she doesn't want the whole school to be told. Try asking her why she thinks you want to tell the school, and go through a typical day at school and see how her diabetes might need to be considered during the day, for example, at mealtimes, PE or exams. If others knew, it would be easier to make adjustments for her diabetes management at these times, or perhaps adjustments could be made in her diabetes management to fit in with school life. You could even ask for a sample timetable to anticipate any changes that need to be made, such as giving less rapid-acting insulin one morning if there is to be an active PE lesson first thing.

Some children decide to use school assembly as a forum to talk about diabetes, others prefer just to tell their class or ask the diabetes specialist nurse to come in.

At the end of this chapter there are some young people's ideas about what would help them in school.

Not many people know [I have diabetes] – it doesn't come up in conversation.

(Janina, 13)

Every time I go to do my injection they come around me and ask me loads of questions...I go out to play and they always ask 'Why are you eating that?...**Why are you eating that?** ...WHY ARE YOU EATING THAT?'

(Aiden, 9)

In the playground you are different from everyone else because you have to eat fruit. They ask you, 'Is there something wrong with you?' It makes you feel different and I am ashamed to say that I am diabetic.

(Amanda, 9)

Some people like to watch me do my injection, but I don't let them because it's gross. Some people say, 'Can you do it again so I can watch?' Then they say, 'Ooh, that's gross'.

(Chantelle, 12)

I got my diabetic nurse to come into school and she took assembly, explaining about Type 1 and 2.

(Kaya, 12)

Q Janie has come home a few times upset saying that she feels different because she has diabetes. She seemed so happy at primary school and now she is withdrawn.

A Some young people with diabetes can feel different. No child wants to be different at school and will not be convinced however many times they are reassured that they are 'special' and 'different'. Who

continued on next page

continued

are you kidding? It's all very well to be different because you have been selected for the Arsenal junior squad. Being different because you have to check your blood sugars, do injections and watch what you eat isn't really that appealing. It is pointless trying to play it down, because there is an element of truth in it. You may find it painful as it may trigger feelings of guilt and blame. However, dismissing your child's feelings may make them feel even more isolated.

Moving from primary to secondary school, and making new friends, is a big step for anyone. Add to that the worries about diabetes in the new school day and it can all be a bit much.

Take a typical school day. If your child is on a twice-daily insulin regimen, having snacks at roughly the same time of day is important. Ideally, all school children should be choosing healthy food options, but the reality is often not ideal. If your child is on a four-times-a-day injection regimen and needing to inject at lunchtime, he or she may be injecting before or after lunch. If it is before lunch they may need to leave class early in order to go to the Medical Room and do their injection and then be at the front of the queue for lunch. If injecting after lunch, they are likely to lose some playtime and miss out on games with their friends.

Having to do blood tests and injections in school can be a hassle and an embarrassment. Having to go into the Medical Room for these occasions makes you stick out like a sore thumb and can make you miss out on things that are going on. Of course they do need to be done, but how sensible it would be if tests and injections could be done in the classroom or at the dinner table without a fuss.

Mum says I'm special because I'm different. I don't want to be different, I just want to be the same as everyone else.

(Amanda, 9)

I'm the only one in my school with diabetes. I sort of feel left out.

(Leo, 10)

At school people were bullying me, saying I had diabetes because I'd eaten too much sugar.

(Chantelle, 12)

I go to the medical room after eating [to do my injection]. Sometimes I get annoyed – it takes ages getting the key then I miss half my playtime.

(Janina, 13)

When I play football, I'm about to score the top goal and it's like 'Aiden, you have to do your blood sugar'...it takes over your life...every thing you do, it interrupts it.

(Aiden, 9)

At school sometimes people say, 'I wish I had diabetes', but they don't really understand what it is. They say 'You're so lucky'. I say, 'When you get it and you have to do an injection every time you eat you'll understand what it's like'.

(Kaya, 12)

Q Melinda's teacher says she keeps getting into fights at school. She never used to. Her school work has gone a bit downhill too. Is it related to her diabetes or is she becoming a moody teenager?

A If Melinda's blood sugars are running high, low, or swinging in between, it may be the cause of mood swings. If you can look at previous blood results on her blood testing machine, it will soon answer that question.

However, it might be worth thinking about whether she is being called names at school. People usually bully because of ignorance, insecurity or because they themselves were bullied previously. Whatever the reason, if it is your child being bullied you are right to

154

A continued

be upset. Being bullied, verbally or physically, is awful. Name calling can be cruel. It is easy to say 'just ignore them' but in reality that is difficult to do. It makes a child ask 'Why me?' There is no easy answer. The only way forward is to talk to and educate everyone concerned.

Similarly, if your child is bullying others, there may be a reason for it; this change in behaviour may be a cry for help.

They saw me do my injection, then they started bullying me so I hit them around the head.
(Leo, 10, who is said to be a troublemaker at school)

On the estate they called me a 'diabetic sweetbag'. I didn't want that to happen again so I kept quiet about my diabetes. Then when I went to secondary school I was the one who would sort out the bullies in the school.
(George, 35)

They stare and call me druggie and weirdo. It's really annoying.
(Darren, 12, who has been getting into fights at school)

Q In Sam's old school they were fantastic with his diabetes and didn't make a fuss about it. In his new school they won't let him do blood tests in the classroom or carry glucose tablets, which makes me worry in case he has a hypo. How can I get school to take diabetes seriously?

A Diabetes is not a 'disability' when it is treated properly and safely. School should be a safe place where you trust your child will be looked after and can get on with their learning.

continued on next page

continued

Your child may be the only one in the school who has diabetes. If you are lucky, the school may have looked after a child with diabetes before and may understand some of the routines. At worst, a teacher may have a relative with Type 2 diabetes and think that your child's diabetes is the same.

Think back to how you felt when your child was diagnosed. That's it – freaked out and scared. Teachers at school are likely to feel a similar way.

Children have different experiences in school depending on the level of knowledge and interest of their teachers. Some teachers just don't understand, or don't want to be involved. The start of this chapter sets out the relevant guidelines and legal standards you should expect. However, having to use this to get your child the care they need may cause a rift between you and the school. It might be better to let your diabetes specialist nurse do the liaising at first, although ultimately you will need to play a large part in providing information.

It can be overwhelming for your child to fight for the right just to do a blood test, eat a snack or do an injection at the right time whilst struggling with the demands of school. This is all unnecessary, and can usually be sorted out pretty easily.

There are a few simple rules to managing diabetes in school. These rules are important to the school because, first, they optimise learning and allow the child to access the curriculum (both low and high blood glucose levels will affect a child's ability to learn) and second, persistently raised blood glucose now may cause complications in the future. No school will want to inhibit a child's future. School will also need a simple explanation about diabetes that your diabetes specialist nurse should be able to provide. You may find it useful to photocopy this chapter to give to school.

Teachers who do not understand about diabetes will not realise how important it is to check blood glucose levels if you feel hypo and to have access to glucose tablets. They need to know that waiting until the end of class can be dangerous.

On the other hand, some teachers may be sympathetic, and think that they are being kind by treating your child differently. They may

A continued

even make diabetes an excuse to let them get away with things that they shouldn't. This will only encourage your child (and their class-mates) to question whether they are the same as everyone else, and give them the idea that they can use diabetes as an excuse to get away with things or get out of things. If you have diabetes it's easy to let it get you out of a difficult or unwanted situation at school. Also, if you are a teacher and show your ignorance, you will lose the child's respect. Neither approach will do your child any favours in the long run, even though everyone may agree that they deserve special treatment.

Parents need to be educated and informed so they can advise school. Paediatric diabetes specialist nurses are there to help parents engage with schools and to draw up a Health Care Plan that will be followed. Raise everyone's expectations of what care should be provided: just because there is some resistance that is no reason not to expect it to happen, for the sake of your child's future. Teachers need information so that they are not frightened of diabetes but know how to act appropriately. This will empower teachers, and help them to tell when a child is using their diabetes as an excuse.

If I say I have to test my blood sugar in class, one teacher says OK...another one completely ignores me.

(Aiden, 9)

This mean maths teacher - if I have to have a Dextrose or do my injection she just says 'No' and I have to have it at the end of the class.

(Darren, 12)

When teachers find out they ask me the same questions. In my first year [of diagnosis], if I was high they'd send me home - it was fun! I can get away with a lot of stuff in school. You get a [disability] band for Thorpe Park-you don't have to queue for rides!

(Janina, 13)

Once in school I was doing my blood test. My tutor was shouting at me, 'Do it anywhere just not here'. I got angry and threw my machine at her. They told the Headteacher. I don't do it in school any more or my injection 'cos the teachers are all moaney. Sometimes when my blood's low they think I'm bunking.

(Kiet, 16)

Q John has glucose tablets and biscuits when his blood glucose is low, and then when it's someone's birthday at school he's not allowed to join in with the sweet things that everyone else is eating. How can I avoid giving him mixed messages? Is this doing him any harm?

A Watching your friends eat treats which are passed in front of you while your salivary glands go into overtime is unfair. Any young person wants to be included, not to be left out, but to be just like everyone else: so it is up to them whether they eat sweet things or not. Eating a little bit of sugary food around snack time won't do any harm, and if they save the rest of their 'loot' for snack time later, or tomorrow, this will show you they understand the problem. Even if they do understand, and still scoff the lot, that's normal child behaviour – and adult behaviour too! This will probably cause high blood glucose and may make them feel unwell, and this may be a good opportunity to talk about food and blood glucose and what to do next time round (see Chapter 5: Food and eating). Feeling at first hand what happens when their blood is high because of a 'sweet load' is not likely to cause any great harm, but may be a curve in the learning process.

It is important that John has access to glucose tablets for hypos, but even these can be tempting if your child thinks they taste delicious. It can also be a problem if others know about them, too.

Children with diabetes understand how important it is to have Dextrose to treat hypos and to eat a snack before, during or after PE. They know because they will have experienced the horrible

continued on next page

A continued

feeling of a hypo. No one who does not have diabetes can know what it feels like to have a hypo. But in school, other children will not understand about hypos and may just see your child's supplies as available snacks. Other children may not understand why your child eats, for example, fruit for snacks and biscuits when they are 'hypo'. It's upsetting to have your snacks stolen: it's not only a snack but also treatment in case of a hypo.

I have a biscuit thief in my school.

(Leo, 10)

I have to eat a snack in the middle of class. I always eat a banana every day at 10. They call me Bananaman and tell me I'm lucky because I get to eat in the middle of class. I just feel embarrassed 'cos everyone is looking at me.

(Amanda, 9)

At birthdays they give out little chocolates...sometimes to tell you the truth I'm a bit peckish so I eat them too.

(Margaret, 12)

They don't understand that you have to do injections four times a day. They just think that you get to eat sugar whenever you want. Other people think I can't eat cake.

(Chantelle, 12)

Q Janine is 10. She wants to go on a school trip next term but is not doing her own injections yet. I have been encouraging her for ages but she just won't do it. The school has asked me if I want to come on the trip but I worry that she will be teased. I don't want her to miss out on the trip.

A School trips can be a challenge for parents. You may not want your child to go. After all, who will look after their diabetes? What if they take the wrong amount or type of insulin? What if...? There are of course lots of 'What ifs' and possibilities for mistakes. However, children who are stopped from going will start to feel they are being punished for having their diabetes, which was not an invited guest in the first place.

The most important thing is your child's safety. It may be possible to train a teacher to do or supervise the injections. However, your child may miss out if they are not willing to learn for themselves. Pushing your child into doing something they don't feel ready for may cause arguments and distress. Gentle persuasion and practice can help, with enough warning.

It might be worth speaking to the class teacher at the beginning of each year to see if any trips are planned. That way you have time to plan ahead – whether it be introducing the idea slowly by meeting other children your child's age with diabetes, practising on oranges, teddies, dolls or on you with 'dry shots' before injecting themselves (see Chapter 4: Injection time). Planning and discussion between school and your diabetes team should make it possible.

What you can do

- **Visit the school** with the paediatric diabetes specialist nurse (or another diabetes team member) soon after your child is diagnosed. Talk to the Head Teacher and any other staff who teach or care for your child. Leave plenty of leaflets for everyone to take away and read. If your child is of preschool age, ask your diabetes team which local schools they have good experiences with, when choosing a school.

■ **Be careful with the tone of your approach.** People respond better to requests than demands. A good approach is to describe what the hospital diabetes team needs to make sure your child stays healthy, with good diabetes control. If your child cannot do their own blood tests and injections, say 'The diabetes team needs the blood glucose tested at lunchtime and an injection given. How can this best be done?' Offer to come and show whoever will be doing it what they need to know in order to feel confident.

■ **Draw up a Health Care Plan.** Do this with your diabetes team; include the times of blood tests and injections, and spell out what action needs to be taken in response to a high or low blood glucose. Go through this with the school, and make sure they have several copies.

■ **Spread the net wide.** The more people you inform and educate at school the better. At a secondary school, try to speak with the Head Teacher, the class teacher, the school nurse, the head of year and all PE staff.

■ **If there is resistance, try again.** Ask your diabetes team to reinforce the message of how important diabetes management is for school performance and minimising the risk of longer-term complications.

If there is still resistance, arrange a meeting with the Head Teacher and a member of the diabetes team. You could give them the legislation summary set out by Diabetes UK and ask how you can work together to implement the Health Care Plan. Ask, rather than tell, the Head Teacher how it could be done. Could someone in school, perhaps a teaching assistant, be trained to do what parents do at home? Does the Local Education Authority need to be approached for extra funding for time to supervise blood tests and injections? Is it necessary to obtain a Statement of Special Educational Needs (which usually apply to children with learning difficulties)?

■ **Stay optimistic.** Try to stay positive and engage with the school. Remember that may be a new experience for the school, too.

Here are some suggestions from young people about what would have made their life in school easier. It just goes to show that if you ask children what they would like, they often have brilliant solutions of their own.

■ **Mark the school register.** Making the diagnosis known on the school register would allow the teacher to be made aware of the diagnosis 'so you don't have to explain yourself every time'. This is particularly relevant in schools with a high staff turnover.

- **Spread information.** The paediatric diabetes specialist nurse should be the first port of call for providing the school with general information about diabetes and specific information about your child. They are often able to go into schools to make contact with teachers directly. Someone needs to decide what is the right kind of information to give to other children in school, and the right amount, and who gives it. This might be your child, a teacher or the specialist nurse.

- **Display positive role models.** One young person wanted her classmates to meet an adult with diabetes so they could see how 'normal' they were. She felt that the diabetes information was best coming from someone with diabetes so that her classmates could directly identify with them and would listen. It might then stop the repetitive diabetes-related questions. However, she did not want to be giving out the information herself. She said, 'I'd like someone who is diabetic and grown up to tell my form what diabetes and insulin is and why I have to take an injection'.

My son is due to start school in September, and so far I've had three meetings to discuss how they are going to 'deal' with him, but we still haven't finalised things. They are being very supportive, but it's just something that other parents don't have to deal with, or worry about. I need to know that when I hand my child over at the start of the day that they will look after him as well as I would - that they will check his blood sugars, and make sure he eats his snack and lunch.

(A mother)

Rachel's view

I can't understand how schools don't allow children do their blood tests and injections at their desk or the dinner table. Clearly this may be difficult for young children for whom it takes longer and needs more checking. However, for the older child who just needs a bit of supervision or can inject themselves, making them leave class early seems to me crazy; they miss class and they look and therefore feel different. Children who can do their injection themselves do not necessarily need to be at the front of the dinner queue and if they need a lunchtime injection could do it in their tummy while at the table. It's Health and Safety regulations gone mad if a child can't do a quick blood test or keep their kit with them.

Clearly, teachers need education and since they may never have encountered diabetes in childhood before, they may either have no knowledge or misinformed preconceptions. It can be dangerous for children to be sent out of class when hypo and not be allowed to carry their blood test and glucose tablets with them. On the other hand, teachers should not be offering up excuses for children to use because of their diabetes. Easy excuses coupled with school policy results in a child with diabetes being separated from the rest of the class both physically and emotionally.

It was probably easier when I was young when there weren't such Health and Safety rules. I always carried my blood testing kit and glucose tablets with me. I did a blood test at my desk and an injection sometimes, although I often chose to do this in private. I needed some quiet, concentration and privacy. My school trusted me and similarly I didn't use my diabetes as an excuse and the teachers didn't offer them up to me, in part I think because I had my kit with me and I could do my blood test if needed.

Information for schools

Diabetes UK and Juvenile Diabetes Research Foundation (JDRF) both provide information leaflets and packs for schools (see www.diabetes. org.uk, www.jdrf.org.uk).

Diabetes UK has produced two documents which can be downloaded from the internet or requested free of charge. The first (*Children with diabetes at school – what all staff need to know*) provides general information about diabetes. The second (*Making all children matter: Support for children with diabetes in schools*) summarises the current legislation regarding management of diabetes in schools.

Diabetes UK, in collaboration with three other charities, has produced *Medical Conditions at School*, a policy resource pack. This gives schools specific information on diabetes, and also guidance on how to produce a medical conditions policy. It is available for school staff to download at www.medicalconditionsatschool.org.uk.

Juvenile Diabetes Research Foundation (JDRF) provides information and support for parents, teachers and children in school, which is available through the website (ww.jdrf.org.uk).

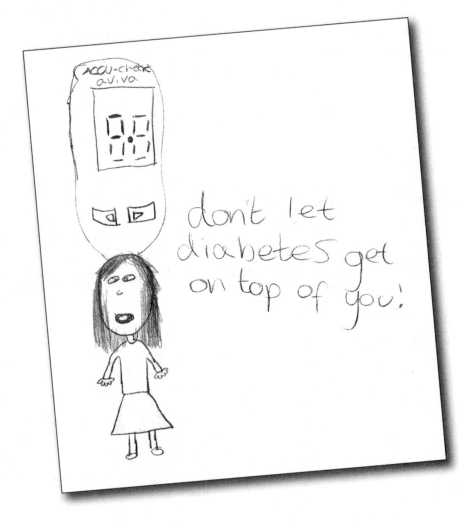

8

Family and friends

When your child is diagnosed with diabetes, so is the whole family. How you relate to each other within the family unit will influence how your child relates to their diabetes. How your child relates to their diabetes, as well as how your family deals with your child's diabetes, will affect you every day, now and in the future.

Family and friends may have preconceptions about diabetes based on one person they knew a long time ago, or on something they heard or read. Children's friends are often unfussed about diabetes, even though their parents may be concerned.

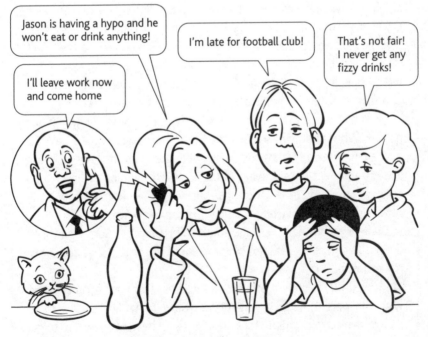

Diabetes affects the whole family

Children often remember one particular thing someone says or does, which stays in their mind. It might be something perfectly innocent but a child can interpret it to give a different meaning than was intended. These seemingly small things can shape a young person's outlook and explain how that individual feels and subsequently behaves.

Previous chapters have focused on how a young person may feel about certain aspects of their diabetes. In this chapter, I have gathered comments from parents, brothers and sisters and friends, as well as from those with diabetes, in the hope of taking a 360-degree view of diabetes within the family unit and beyond. As I was doing so, many people expressed surprise at how others viewed them, until it was discussed. It just goes to show that no one knows what someone else thinks of us until we ask the question, and listen to the answer.

Case 1

A mother's view

On a good day it's just another thing about Sam. He's bright, loves reading, plays rugby with his dad, has diabetes, and seems to own more toy tanks and fighter planes than any other boy. Diabetes means that Sam has grown up faster than other children in some respects. He's strong and independent. He's incredibly brave. He knows what a pancreas is. It's only diabetes – it's not like he's got a terminal illness, or a mental illness – my husband says its eczema with needles.

On a bad day it's utterly horrible. I hate it. I really, really hate it. It's not fair. What did my beautiful little boy do to deserve this? I can't let him go. It's caused heartache, anger, deep hurt and feelings of being less than perfect in my 7-year-old boy. He's too young to have to go through some of these emotions. And yet, when he comes out the other side he will be stronger, braver, and more secure.

Diabetes has made me think about my position as Sam's mother. I am not in control of his life. I play my part, but some things are out of my control.

Every time I drop him off somewhere I have to have a 'quick word' with the parent, carer or organiser. I have to let go, trust him to recognise his symptoms, to look after himself. I have to allow him to get

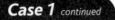

Case 1 *continued*

it wrong. I have to allow someone else to look after him and for him or her to get it wrong too. I have to stop myself from becoming controlling and neurotic.

When do I tell him that he can't join the armed services? His father was in the Royal Navy, his grandfather in the Army and his great-grandfather before him. He longs to join the RAF. He's only seven – but one day he will learn the truth. Who will tell him? Who will pick him up?

Who will look after him when he is 80? Will somebody check his blood sugar for him? Am I doing a good job? Am I too harsh some-times? Should I cut a bit of slack or keep on and on at him – have you checked your blood, what have you had to eat, have you had your snack? What can I do to help him more? What really annoys him about the way I handle his diabetes?

Discussion

You may recognise many of the feelings Sam's mother expresses. Sam, with his family, has to manage day to day with the ins and outs of a diabetes regimen. Sam's mum feels that she is not in control of his life because of his diabetes. She feels that she is hassling Sam about his diabetes, knows she needs to, but also worries about annoying him.

Sam's priorities will be different from his mum's. Sam will be much more interested in his school friends and upcoming birthday parties than his diabetes. However, if asked, he may already sense some of his mum's worries. At 7 years of age, Sam probably does need support and reminding about various aspects of his diabetes such as snacks and checking his blood glucose, as well as other non-diabetes related things like brushing his teeth and taking the right books to school.

Sam's mother has a 'quiet word' with Sam's carer or organiser, hoping he will be looked after safely, but without a fuss. Yet all the time they are apart she is worrying about him. The questions that she wants to ask Sam clearly come from her love for him and her worry about him, now and in the future. I wonder why she does not ask them to Sam directly. I wonder whether many of you reading this book do not directly ask your child those burning questions. Perhaps it is fear of the answer, or fear that you or your child may be upset by the question, or anxiety about introducing an idea into your child's mind. Sam's mother told me that she hasn't asked Sam because she worries that if he knew she was thinking these thoughts he might start worrying himself, and discussing them may remind him of the negative aspects of his diabetes and make him dwell on them. She worries in the hope that Sam doesn't have to.

Perhaps by reading this book you are hoping to find the hidden clues as to how your child feels. The easiest way to find out is to ask. Your child may not want to discuss it there and then, but showing you are interested and have considered the question may allow the subject to come up at a later time. Not talking about things does not stop a child, or adult, thinking about them; it just stops them talking about them.

A selection of parents told me what diabetes means to them. Many of you may relate to these feelings and by reading them I hope you will feel that you are not alone.

A life change for my child and all those who interact with her

Diabetes fits in around us

Being careful

The spontaneity of life has gone and we do not have the carefree attitude that we once had

Everything has to be planned, organised and disciplined

We're all a lot more healthy now

I don't relax as much as I did

I used to have a lovely small Radley handbag. Now I have a big handbag stuffed full of juice cartons, Dextrose and bags of breadsticks!

Sometimes I feel isolated

Other people's ignorance and attitude

I've lost my healthy child

What parents say about their child's diabetes (continued facing page)

‘Change in personality’

‘My other children have to suffer too’

‘Injustice’

‘Inconvenience’

‘Hypos are stressful’

‘Responsibility’

‘It's all a big issue’

‘Diabetes is messing up our lives’

‘Will they lead a 'normal' life?’

‘I feel angry about having this 'thing' in our lives. It's a bit like having a monster in the house – you lock it away in a cupboard and try to forget about it, but every so often it comes out and bites you.’

‘It's difficult getting babysitters’

‘It's made me appreciate my daughter growing up to be healthy and fulfilled, without letting the diabetes get in her way’

What parents say about their child's diabetes

Case 2

A brother remembers

Introducing Guy, 33

Diabetes was a part of all of our lives from an early age. It still is. We've always had sugar-free drinks in the house and lots of fruit. It has set me up for living a healthier lifestyle.

Before my sister was diagnosed all I remember was her drinking gallons of water from the tap in the kitchen. She was taken into hospital. I remember Mum and Dad hugging when they got the news. It really hit home for me when all four of us were with the doctor and she was crying when she was told she couldn't eat normal sweets again. I felt bad for her. Once she had a hypo and went downstairs to get an orange juice. She fell down the stairs

continued on next page

Case 2 *continued*

because of her low blood sugar. It was the last time she was allowed to get her own orange juice when she was low. I had to go to Maths Club early because she had to go to hospital. I was worried about her.

I am so proud of what she's done and the battles she's overcome. For a while diabetes dominated her life but now she handles it well and doesn't let it stop her doing anything. She works and plays hard, has good friends and knows how to have fun. She looks fantastic and is incredibly fit.

I still worry now though that she might not have as long a life as she might otherwise have had, that she might lose her eyesight and limbs. I'm lucky that I don't have diabetes.

Discussion

Like many brothers and sisters, Guy remembers details about his sister being diagnosed with diabetes and certain key events, such as her first big hypo. He watched silently and took it all in. He built up worries which are still present, even though he rationally knows that she is well.

Guy feels lucky that he doesn't have diabetes, implying that his sister is unlucky that she does. This is a burden he still carries. During all the noise that accompanies diagnosis, hypos and injections, brothers and sisters also watch and take it all in. Some worries may be based on their interpretations of events that are not a reality. If they are not explored they may lie dormant, breeding anxieties which may influence that relationship.

Case 3

A young person's view of how their diabetes affects other family members

Introducing Jason, 27, diagnosed aged 7

Mum never forced me to do anything. Obviously she was worried about my diabetes but she never conveyed it to me. Even now she hates the thought of me going out, getting drunk and collapsing

---

somewhere. She rarely tells me. When I was growing up she kept an eye on me but never made it clear that she was.

When I was first diagnosed we all converted to low fat and sugar-free. The only time I'd have anything different was when I was on a plane flight – it was really embarrassing and disgusting.

I have two sisters, both older than me. I was never treated any differently nor made to feel different. They were always jealous that I could eat what I wanted to eat. They'd say 'It's not fair' when I'd be eating biscuits when I was hypo.

Discussion

Jason seems to have a healthy attitude towards his diabetes now, although he does acknowledge that he has felt awkward at times. He says that he was treated no differently to the rest of the family. However, just by having diabetes he would have been treated differently. His sisters were envious of his hypo 'treats'. Like many young people who see someone eating food when they are hypo, they think this is special treatment. However, they will never experience the blood tests, injections and hypos themselves, first hand, only second hand when they may get woken in the night whilst their brother or sister with diabetes is checked on. Brothers and sisters who never have hypos but who are also not allowed certain foods may then end up feeling punished themselves.

However hard you try, brothers and sisters will never be treated the same; but you can only do your best. Having a 'treat' when you feel unwell with a hypo, compared to a 'treat' when you feel fine is not the same, and is not fair.

Jason was diagnosed at 7 years old. Despite his age, he was always aware of how his mum worried, and still does. Most young people are aware of how you feel, to a lesser or greater degree, even if you think you are hiding it well. It is much better to talk about the feelings that both of you have. If you can't do this with your child, talking with someone else in the same position, such as another parent or a healthcare professional who understands diabetes, can help relieve some stress and feelings of isolation.

For many young people, diabetes is not such a big deal. It is probably more of an issue for you than for them. Being a good parent means that you will worry about your children forever and the responsibilities will never go away. You don't need me to tell you that having a child brings rewards, like seeing them getting married, making you grandparents and loving you back. You owe it to yourself and your children to ease your own burden and guilt otherwise you will carry these as well as the day-to-day worries which is not good for any of you.

Case 4

A young person and her friends discuss diabetes
Introducing Lizzie, 27, diagnosed aged 8

In the beginning diabetes was easy. Mum cooked food, I was into exercise and my friends weren't bothered. I always worried and still do worry that my brother was left out. I was always congratulated about managing my diabetes, which wasn't an achievement like running or doing well in Maths. He was left out.

When I went to secondary school there were lots of questions about my diabetes. Friends didn't make a fuss about my diabetes but their parents did. Some were really worried and called Mum for reassurance. It made me feel different.

As I got older, my diabetes became more of a focus in my life. If anything went wrong, in my head it was all because of my diabetes in some way. The tangle with emotion and food interplayed strongly with my diabetes. There wasn't a lot of room for anyone else, as my relationship with my diabetes was such a strong presence. Also, I thought that no one else could really understand how I felt. I kept my feelings to myself and put on a brave front, but inside I felt alone.

At college I used to hide the fact that I had diabetes from everyone, including boyfriends. Then when they'd find out, I'd give a curt sharp reply and they wouldn't mention it again. I'd hate the curiosity and questioning that my diabetes would bring, and also the fact that everyone was always so impressed with how I seemed to be dealing with it. I'd think, it's not like I had any choice about being diagnosed, I have no choice but to get on with it. I'd wonder why they wanted to

Case 4 *continued*

know so much about my diabetes, it made me feel that they weren't interested in me, just my diabetes.

I was always scared that I would be rejected because I had diabetes, but the reality is that the only person who has ever rejected me because of my diabetes is me.

I have had to slowly cut the ties I have with my diabetes and make it less of the main focus in my life. It's too easy to use diabetes as an excuse or crutch.

I now have friends who have diabetes. They are incredibly important to me, as they understand what I go through with my diabetes – the significance and insignificance of the role it plays in my life. We don't need to explain it to each other. We are members of an invitation-only club, one that of course none of us really want to be members of if we didn't have to.

Charlotte and Debbie have been friends of Lizzie since she was 4 years old.

Charlotte

I remember Lizzie suddenly disappearing from primary school. She was away for about a week. A day or so before she was due back, the teacher told us all that she had diabetes and that she was fine but she was in hospital doing what she had to do. They made it clear that she was healthy and it wasn't life-threatening, but that she wasn't coming back as the same person as she would have to do special things.

Things were fine at primary school. Diabetes was just something Lizzie had to do and she just got on with it. I knew if she came round to my house she'd have to wear slippers inside so she didn't hurt her feet.

One class in primary school when the regular teacher was off and there was a supply teacher, Lizzie went off to eat a banana and then started being told off by the supply teacher. We were all trying to tell the teacher that Lizzie had to eat a banana. The teacher was so apologetic. We were all protective of Lizzie 'cos that's what Lizzie had to do.

continued on next page

Case 4 *continued*

On a school trip I was put with Lizzie in a special corridor room, when everyone else was in dormitories. We had midnight feasts on Lizzie's diabetic sweets that she was allowed to keep with her!

I remember at primary school we went to someone's birthday party. We all ate jelly and ice-cream, but Lizzie was given something different. She was really frustrated. I knew she didn't want to be seen as different, it made her stick out like a sore thumb. She didn't not want to be the same as everyone else. After that I went home and told Mum and Dad that if Lizzie comes round, you have to give her what we have. I said, 'You have to give Lizzie ice-cream. She might not eat it all, but you have to give her the same thing we eat'. A lot of parents assumed that diabetes meant that Lizzie couldn't eat sugar.

Sometimes when she'd get a new blood test machine she'd show me. I was always interested.

Then there was a time when she didn't want to talk about it. She went to university and wanted to be normal. She saw university as a fresh start and didn't want anyone to know she had diabetes. We lost touch a bit during that time. I think she was worried about me meeting her new friends and giving away her secret. I was a reminder. I was worried that she was hiding it. Inevitably when friends did find out she got upset when they asked questions and she was defensive about it. She felt an outsider and just wanted to fit in.

Debbie

I was at primary school with Lizzie when she developed diabetes. She was about eight or nine. I remember her being away for a couple of weeks, coming back and having been diagnosed with something. It meant all of a sudden she had to have a routine to follow but it didn't seem to be too difficult. I was aware her energy would go low sometimes. Up until a few years ago, Lizzie didn't talk about her diabetes. At some point she was allowed to eat chocolate. I noticed it and thought, that's good.

Discussion

For Lizzie, her diabetes has been a large part of her daily life. As for her friends, they have always known it is there, but their friendship with Lizzie has little to do with her diabetes. But Lizzie felt different even though her friends did not see her that way.

Charlotte and Debbie, like I expect most of Lizzie's friends, saw her as a whole person. However, when Lizzie went to friends' houses, their parents were inevitably preoccupied with Lizzie's diabetes. Friends knew it wasn't a big deal, but then they spent time with Lizzie every day. Friends' parents will remember how diabetes used to be managed, and know about all the problems it brought. It is clear from Charlotte that even though she and Lizzie didn't talk much about diabetes, she knew that Lizzie didn't want to be treated differently. Charlotte tried to educate her parents and teachers. You can feel how protective Charlotte feels about Lizzie's treatment by others even though it was not discussed between them at the time. It just goes to show how we all, no matter what age, pick up on the feelings of others around us.

Diabetes became an issue for Lizzie, not so much because of the diabetes itself, but because of other people's reaction to it. It is easy to see why Lizzie became introspective. In this situation, it is understandable to keep things to yourself if 'no one understands me'.

Q I am always either organising snacks, supervising injections, doing blood tests or writing them down. I feel like my relationship has changed with my son and I have become a 'diabetic mother' but my husband is still just 'dad'. How can I stop becoming 'the worrier'?

A When your child is diagnosed, all the focus will be on them. You may feel that you begin to relate in a different way with your child. You may have become the nag, worrier, administrator of painful injections and blood tests. On the other hand, the change may not necessarily all be negative as it may bring you all closer together, and provide an opportunity to have a healthier lifestyle. I hope you will agree from reading this book that encouraging your child and

continued on next page

continued

being interested in how your child feels about their diabetes is important. It is also important that you and your other children get the opportunity to talk about how you feel, even if it is hard in the beginning. Your own feelings, as well as those of your child, will affect all of your interactions.

You may find that one parent ends up doing more of the diabetes care than the other, just like in some families it is always one parent who does more of the telling off or more of the ironing. It's probably not fair on either of you and provides plenty of opportunity for your children to play one of you off against the other!

I wonder why your partner is not 'doing their fair share'? Perhaps they do not like being reminded of the suffering they feel their child is going through; it may even provoke feelings in them of the guilt and anger they feel about their child's diabetes. Or maybe they weren't around at the beginning and now just feel out of their depth. Everyone, parents and children alike, will make mistakes at some point. Some mistakes will be minor, such as forgetting a snack, but others will seem like huge cock-ups, like giving the evening insulin dose twice. While it may sound ridiculous, actually this mistake is easy to make, but is absolutely terrifying once the mistake has been discovered. Some parents in this situation will be put off getting involved ever again, or their partner may not let them, which is punishing them twice over. Even adults with diabetes sometimes forget they have done their insulin and do it twice or miss it completely and under- or overtreat hypos. Before you get too cross, ask yourself when you last forgot to take the Pill or a dose of antibiotics.

Whatever it is, there will be a reason why your partner is not getting involved. If you are finding all the diabetes care too much to cope with on your own, sit down when things are calm and work it out, get over it and on with it, otherwise not only will you stay angry but your children will pick up on it too.

We've all got used to it together.

(Margaret, 12)

Mum helps me with my injection when I can't be bothered. Dad just reminds me. He asks me to leave a note to say I've done it. Mum goes on at me but Dad lets me be independent. I know that Mum is trying to care for me in a way. Mum uses my diabetes as an excuse. She prefers my brother. He gets more chocolate than me. She says that I'm diabetic and he needs to put on weight. I know he's a bit thin but I think it's a bit unfair. I might have a yoghurt and he'll have a chocolate mousse. I get angry. I don't say much, then I go and scream in my pillow.

(Summer, 13)

I used to hate the reminders from Mum to do my blood test and injection. She would always say to me as I walked out the door to play, 'Have you got your glucose tablets?' At a young age it used to drive me mad. The constant reminders to me felt like being hassled by my parents non-stop. I used to stay out of sight of the house or later than agreed, purposely to wind them up and of course worrying my Mum that I had had a hypo. Even when I got older my parents would shout up to my bedroom, 'Do your injection, dinner will be soon'!

(Rebecca, 35)

Q **I worry that Jamie's brother, who doesn't have diabetes, feels pushed aside, left out and that I don't give him as much attention.**

A A diagnosis of diabetes in the family involves everyone in that family. Around diagnosis the child with diabetes has so much attention that there's not a lot of time to think about how it is affecting you, your other children and any extended family. Brothers and sisters can often feel left out. They may feel upset for their brother or sister who has diabetes and helpless, but surprisingly, they may also feel jealous of the attention. At other times they may be cross that they have to change their routine just to suit the diabetes.

continued on next page

continued

Here are some comments from children and adults who do not have diabetes, about their brothers and sisters who do.

'I feel bad for her that she can't eat sweets'

'We have to eat mealtimes at set times, then I can't go out to play'

'It's a nuisance'

'Sometimes diabetes keeps me up at night'

'Sometimes I have to go to the hospital in the night with him'

'It's not fair'

'I was worried when she was taken into hospital'

'She gets more treats than me'

'What about me?'

'I miss having sweets too'

'Sometimes I feel sad'

'Sometimes I feel angry'

'Sometimes I feel lonely'

'In RE I prayed to God they'd find a cure for diabetes'

'I'd break my arm to find a cure for diabetes'

'They keep checking on him'

'There's always Dextrose and Lucozade in the house'

'I've got to stay in and stay in line'

'They get all the attention from Mum and Dad'

'I have to get up early at weekends'

'I worry he might die'

'Sometimes diabetes stops me from doing things'

'Friends don't know enough about diabetes'

What siblings say about diabetes

'I understand why he gets moody but it doesn't help – I still don't like it'

'Sometimes she uses her diabetes to get out of doing chores'

'Sometimes I get told off for things that aren't my fault'

'I'm worried that I might get diabetes too'

'I get more sweets now whenever they have a hypo'

'At school people ask me 'What's it like to live with someone with diabetes?''

'I'd like to make diabetes go away'

'It hurts me when he cries'

'We're all more healthier now'

'They get more sleepovers than me'

'I feel good when she's brave'

'He doesn't like needles'

'Other parents don't understand so we all get left out'

'Mum and Dad get stressed because of diabetes'

What siblings say about diabetes

My brother is eighteen months younger than me. It was difficult for him. I got more attention because of my diabetes. He's always felt he had something to live up to. I used to ask, why doesn't he have diabetes? It didn't feel fair.

(Katherine, 30)

It wasn't fair that Susie always came first but we had no choice. We always worried about her brother not getting as much attention. We never talked about it with him as we didn't want to put the idea of him feeling sad or left out into his mind.

(Susie's mum)

Q Is it fair to treat siblings differently?

A Even putting diabetes aside, of course it isn't fair. Add diabetes to the mix and things start to get more complicated.

The issue of equality in treatment between siblings often centres on food as well as attention. Many of you may feel that your other children, who don't have diabetes, are made to suffer because their brother or sister does. You may want to sneak them a bar of chocolate and make a pact to 'keep it our secret'. But surely it is just as cruel to the child with diabetes to deny them treats as it is to the brother or sister who doesn't have diabetes. This is why the modern diabetes regimens should be incorporating a healthy diet. However, if your child is on a twice- or three-times-a-day regimen, it is less flexible in terms of food and you may need to follow certain food rules.

Here are a few options.

- You could treat them both/all the same, which may cause resentment and 'It's not fair'.
- You could pretend to treat them the same but actually not do so, which will encourage your child without diabetes to see your child who does have it differently; consciously or subconsciously this may affect their relationship.
- You could change the house to sugar-free and healthier options. This is fine as long as you don't keep treats to torment your child with diabetes in the house and can stick to this without going to the corner shop for Mars bars when everyone has gone to bed for yourself to snack on and for your other child's lunchbox.
- You could free yourself up by going onto a more flexible insulin regimen, such as a four-times-a-day regimen or an insulin pump, both of which allow more freedom with food.

If you were to follow this last option, your child could eat what others are eating and take this into account with the insulin dose. You could give some extra fast-acting insuin and can allow ice-cream at the end of a meal. Of course, whatever course you follow you will be treating your child with diabetes differently – after all, no one would ever conceivably want to have to take an injection every time

A *continued*

they eat. However, until there are more practical management regimens to make life with diabetes easier, this is the best of a bad situation. Insulin pumps get around many of these problems, but they are not ideal or practical for everyone (see Chapter 4: Injection time, for further explanation of the use of an insulin pump).

My sister was diagnosed after me. It wasn't a shock, I just hoped she could cope with it. I thought it was a new friend after being alone. She feels how I feel. Now I don't have to see her eat sweets and enjoy life.

(Daniel, 17)

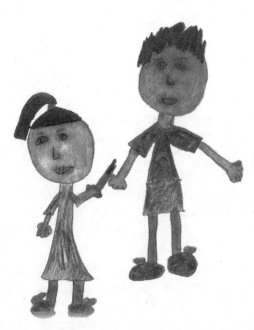

A younger sister drew this picture and writes: 'On my picture I am doing my brother's injection. I hate having injections so I'm glad I haven't got diabetes. But I love my brother a lot and hopefully he loves me, but Mum tells me where to put it and I do it.'

My brother used to get all the attention. When I became diabetic the focus was on me. His mealtimes became my mealtimes and my snacks became his. My brother suffered. All the nice things he would have got, he got denied.

(Ruth, 38)

Q **What should I tell my child's new friends and their parents?**

A This decision has got to come from your child, not from you. As in Case 4 above, often other children understand what is going on better than their parents. Many of your child's friends' parents will have old-fashioned ideas about diabetes and may think they are doing the right thing when it comes to certain food choices or making 'helpful comments', which reinforce the isolation your child may feel.

It would be a good idea to speak to your child's friends' parents about diabetes. That will help when it comes to parties and sleepovers. It will also help prevent the 'useful' and frequently incorrect comments they might be telling their children, such as 'you can't eat sugar', asking if you still have to give injections, or that your child must have eaten too much sugar when they were younger. After all, when children make comments about diabetes to your child, they are likely to come from other children or their parents. It just reflects the wider circle of ignorance that needs addressing.

'Does that mean you have to eat loads of Mars bars?' has been the most applied phrase in the last 20 years.

(Martina, 28)

When I eat something a bit sweet, they say 'You're not meant to eat that!'

(Summer, 13)

Some people have prehistoric ideas about diabetes - like Type 1 is worse than Type 2. The other one is that you can't eat sweets or chocolates.

(Rebecca, 35)

When even the medical profession act surprised and say 'You don't look diabetic, you look so healthy', I think, 'Do you expect it to be tattooed across my forehead? And I am healthy, I just have to inject four times a day.

(Katherine, 30)

My friends ALWAYS want to see me doing my injection. I went on a trip with my school once. I was doing my injection and one girl was staring, then another said, 'Oh do it again I wanted to see'.

(Chantelle, 12)

When I say I have to do injections some people say, 'You must be really severely affected then'. It just shows how little they know about it.

(Susie, 24)

What you can do

■ **Change food habits for everyone.** After all, the whole family is affected by a diagnosis of diabetes. It may be a great opportunity for everyone as far as your food choices at home are concerned. Find a healthy routine, one that works for your family. For example, you could have a 'treats drawer' that you can all choose something from once or twice a week. Don't forget to keep it locked during the rest of the week, though!

- **Start talking.** This is easier said than done. You might need some help with this, from you diabetes team or other parents in the same situation.

- **Talk to friends' parents.** If your child will let you, you and your child could explain to your children's friends and their parents about diabetes and what it means for your child. They may not know anything about diabetes, or they may have old-fashioned and outdated ideas about what diabetes is and how it is managed.

- **Think about brothers and sisters.** They need as much attention as your child with diabetes. This needs to be balanced out, as attention to treat a hypo will not be the same as attention given by going to an adventure park.

- **Go on a family weekend** organised by Diabetes UK. These enjoyable breaks really help the whole family (see Appendix for contact details).

Rachel's view

Jean-Paul Sartre wrote: 'hell is other people'. For me, this perfectly sums up diabetes. If the child were to be left to their diabetes, things would be easier. However, 'other people', even with the best of intentions, put in their twopence-worths, making comments or reacting in ways that cause harm. I certainly took on board particular comments when I was growing up, sometimes from people I hardly knew. For example, when they found out I had diabetes, the reaction was always, 'Oh poor you'. I never wanted people to pity me or treat me differently because of my diabetes, and that made me want to write this book. I could bear it no longer and felt I had to speak out for children with diabetes, then and now.

Many of my worries about other people's reactions to my diabetes are unfounded; they were based on one or two comments that stayed with me, such as from a parent's friends, one boyfriend who used my diabetes as an excuse to end our relationship, and some doctors' ignorance. So it became easier not to let on I had diabetes. However, I don't feel the same now. I must tell, in order to educate others that diabetes is just one extra thing about me I need to do something about. I don't make insulin so I need to replace it.

I always carry the worries my parents and my brother have about my diabetes. However much I tell them I am fine, they always worry. Sometimes it is nice but sometimes it is also an extra burden that I have to carry.

Other people are at most impressed, indifferent or unknowledgeable about diabetes. The only time it has influenced my relationship with them has been in the past when I allowed it to happen. Diabetes is only as big a deal as people make it. So now I practise what I preach.

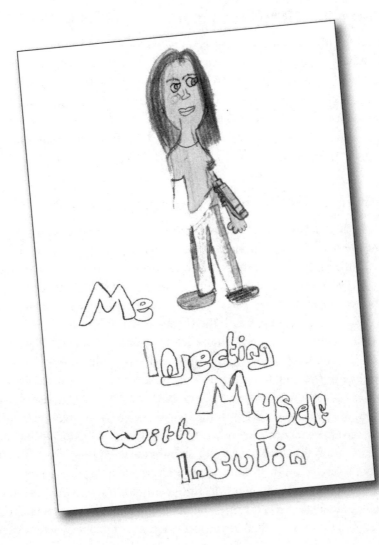

The teenage years

What happens to blood glucose levels in puberty?

Tighter blood glucose levels seem to be harder to maintain during puberty. Some of this can be explained by the increase in certain body chemicals (hormones) that are released by the body into the bloodstream that are necessary for growth and which also push up blood glucose levels. Increasing independence and teenage issues, such as risk-taking behaviours, wanting to fit in, eating junk food and the desire to be thin can also affect blood glucose control.

Can you drink alcohol if you have diabetes?

The medical answer is yes. Alcohol affects everyone differently, but in someone with diabetes it needs to be figured out carefully what alcohol does to the body. It will be affected by how much food is eaten, the quantity and strength of alcohol, and whether the alcoholic drink has carbohydrate in it or not. Parents and teenagers also need to be aware of the risk of hypoglycaemia with the effects of alcohol.

Some drinks containing alcohol will also contain sugar and will push up blood glucose levels. However, alcohol itself also reduces blood glucose levels by not allowing new glucose to be produced from the liver. Alcohol can affect brain functioning so that in some people their awareness of hypo symptoms can be blunted; a tipsy individual may forget to give their insulin injection. Experimenting safely, with regular blood testing during and after drinking alcohol, is the only way for an individual to know what effect the alcohol is having on their blood glucose levels and on their awareness.

Most people with diabetes do not give extra insulin with alcoholic drinks and will eat an extra snack before going to bed; however, this must be tailored to the individual. If you are in a group of people when drinking it is a good idea for someone else in the group to know about diabetes and for you to wear a medical identity necklace or bracelet just in case you have a hypo. The hypo effects of alcohol can last until the next day.

How do drugs affect diabetes?

'Recreational' drugs are illegal but still readily available. Their effect really depends on the type of drug as well as the individual. Some drugs affect appetite, activity levels and awareness of hypoglycaemia symptoms.

Is it safe to drive if you have diabetes?

It is safe to drive if you have good hypo awareness, and are prepared to test your blood glucose level before driving, and always have something readily available to treat a hypo in the car. By law, anyone with diabetes treated by insulin must inform DVLA. Your must self-declare the control and management of your condition and must consent to DVLA making medical enquiry of your doctor, where DVLA thinks it is necessary. If DVLA identifies a possible risk to safe driving on the basis of your honest declaration about your condition, they will contact your own doctor for a report. This ensures that those whose condition is currently a risk are not licensed until better control is attained. Your driving licence needs to be renewed every three years.

When you are driving, it is advisable to stop every one to two hours for a break anyway, and if you are feeling tired you should check your blood glucose level, as tiredness can be mistaken for being hypo or hyper, and vice versa.

Currently those treated with insulin in the UK can drive vehicles under 3.5 tonnes on a 3-year licence. It is prohibited to drive anything over 7.5 tonnes which includes heavy goods vehicles and any passenger-carrying vehicles. To drive a vehicle (excluding a passenger-carrying vehicle) between 3.5 and 7.5 tonnes requires a special medical application and a yearly licence renewal (there is more detail on this in Chapter 10).

Introduction to the cases

For many parents of young children with diabetes, the teenage years are a frightening prospect. Maybe you remember your own and wonder how you would have coped with having diabetes as well as all the other trials of being a teenager. Perhaps you have heard that adolescence with diabetes can be a difficult time, with the pressures and temptations it can bring, coupled with the potential for difficult blood glucose control. You may worry about losing control of your child's routine, your teenager slipping away from you, and want to know what to do. Many of you will just want your child to be able to achieve the right balance of freedom as you did without any disastrous consequence on their diabetes.

While for some young people with diabetes the teenage years can be a difficult time, it is by no means the same for everyone. Whenever someone is asked if they have a story to share, many remember the difficult times. It is worth remembering this as you read the cases in this chapter, many of which paint a frightening picture for parents. These cases bring up issues you may need to deal with, but many young people pass through the teenage years smoothly with a series of checks and balances, and some guidance from you.

Case 1

Skipping injections

Introducing George, 35, diagnosed aged 9

As a teenager I kept my bloods high. I was going out with friends. Mum asked me questions and I gave her the right answers. The hospital turned around and said 'Look after yourself or you'll lose your eyesight and your legs will fall off.' I smoked from the age of 11, drank alcohol and did drugs. Being diabetic didn't make any difference. I was doing what everyone else did. I just wanted to go out and be like everyone else. I was missing my injections, maybe taking one in the morning and one in the evening. I hated being in DKA [diabetic ketoacidosis] because I hated hospitals. I just wanted to be going out with friends.

When I was 12 to 17, I had bad thrush on my penis and I was too embarrassed to say anything about it. I didn't know it at the time but I found out later that it was because of my high blood sugars.

Discussion

The teenage years, the time of transition between childhood and adulthood, can be challenging, and this is particularly so for teenagers with diabetes. As you read through this chapter, which deals with some very challenging probems, it is important to remember that the teenage years don't have to be a nightmare.

It's normal at this time to explore, and experiment with, the outside world as well as one's own body. If you have diabetes as well, that adds another dimension. Some teenagers with diabetes want to do what other teenagers do, and more. They have more tools to experiment with and more issues to think about. For example, a young person with diabetes may have been told that they must never miss an injection as it is life saving. A teenager may miss an injection; it may be part of their self-exploration, experimenting, or forgetfulness when on a night out, or as part of denying their condition. They may not want to inject when they are on a night out or in front of their friends. If they miss an injection they may feel 'a bit grotty' but they will survive it. They may then realise that they can get away without an injection if needs be. They may even feel that their parents and diabetes team have lied to them when they said injections were essential. Another missed injection doesn't have huge consequences either, and soon it becomes normal to miss an injection here or there. Their body may get used to the feeling of experiencing high blood glucose levels. Running high also avoid embarrassing sweaty hypos in front of potential boyfriends or girlfriends. Sometimes what also happens is that a young person misses the odd injection here and there. If this is before puberty or during the honeymoon phase (when some of the body's own insulin is still being made, usually within a couple of years after diagnosis), they may just feel a bit tired and thirsty. However, continuing the same behaviour outside the honeymoon phase and as the pubertal hormones kick in sends the blood glucose levels really high and ketones start being produced causing diabetic ketoacidosis and hospital admission. It's the same behaviour but with a different outcome, which can be confusing.

George wasn't bothered about the warnings of complications. He wanted to make diabetes as small a part of his life as possible. I wonder if someone tried to shock George into keeping better blood glucose levels by threatening him with the risk of complications. It didn't work, and it may even have caused him to deny his diabetes even more.

Teenagers can often only see the short term; 20 years seems like a lifetime away: it will never come. You and your diabetes team will be more interested in the risks of longer-term complications. (See Chapter 6:

Hyperglycaemia, ketoacidosis and complications.) George just wanted to be out with his friends. However, poor blood glucose control can make diabetes a bigger issue than it need be because high and swinging blood glucose levels mean you won't feel as well as you could, and you can do less.

Missing injections during the teenage years is probably the worst time to do it, since insulin requirements go up during puberty as body chemicals (hormones) are released to promote growth. Even when someone is taking injections regularly, blood glucose results can be unpredictable. If they start missing injections as well, blood glucose levels may be completely erratic.

George wanted to be 'normal' and that meant doing what those without diabetes did, and probably more. George, just like anyone with diabetes, did not look different, but he felt it, and that is reflected in his behaviour. The chances are that other factors were in play and it would be too easy solely to blame his diabetes for his behaviour; but it is an important factor that needs to be considered and managed in the 'rebellious child', the one who would be too easy to give up on.

Case 2

Experimenting as a teenager
Introducing Katherine, 30, diagnosed aged 9

I started rebelling when I was 13. I was going through puberty and my bloods were high all the time. I had heavy periods and high blood sugars every month. I was sent to a gynaecologist. It pissed me off that no one could say what the problem was. I got really frustrated.

Then I started to binge eat. It started with satsumas. I would eat 20 at once. It progressed to ice-cream and then to other things. It started off as wanting to see what would happen to my blood sugars. I also experimented by giving extra insulin and then having a big hypo. At that stage everything to do with diabetes was about food. Everybody watched what I was eating.

It took me a while to realise I could give extra insulin and eat more. The doctors and nurses at the hospital didn't tell me that, I figured it out. I knew more than they did.

Case 2 *continued*

When I was about 13, I was in and out of hospital over a 6-month period, in diabetic ketoacidosis. I would binge, be high and then become ketotic. I'd still give the same dose of insulin I usually gave but it wasn't enough for the 12 hours of continuous eating I'd do. There was a bit of one-upmanship with the doctors. I was getting my own back. I had this [diabetes] and I could use it to my own advantage. I didn't like being in hospital, but it was better than school. It was like, 'You can't force me to go to school'. No one at school ever questioned me being off, because of my diabetes.

In hospital, when no one was looking, I'd get out of bed, go to the snack machine, eat chocolate, throw away the packet and go back to bed. Then they'd do my blood sugar and I'd be high. My consultant couldn't work out why and he even wrote a case study about me.

When I moved school I was happier and I stopped bingeing to excess.

Discussion

When you are a teenager it is natural to want to try things that are forbidden and to take risks. For many, having diabetes can make you feel as if you are not in control of your own body. Taking risks can be proof that you feel 'normal'. However, just as in Katherine's case, if the experimenting happens alongside diabetes it can have harmful effects. Katherine had been told to eat certain foods when she was growing up, and when she was a teenager insulin doses and food portion sizes were fixed. She wanted to see what would happen if she broke the rules. She found that, guess what, she could get away with it! Suddenly she felt in control of her body even though it was going haywire with wildly swinging blood glucose levels. Katherine no doubt thought her doctors were a bit stupid, not advising her to change her insulin doses with food as is recommended these days. Katherine started to play a dangerous game to regain power over her own body that she felt she had lost.

Even with today's insulin regimens, giving insulin when you eat is still too regimented a lifestyle for some, and it may be easier to just miss injections completely. It can also feel like an impositon and give a young person the fuel to rebel, fight back and get one over against their own body.

Katherine started to binge eat and she says this was initially an experiment to see what would happen to her blood glucose levels. Fortunately, this resolved when she felt happier in herself when she moved to a new school. However for others, missing injections may also become a tool used to control their weight (see Chapter 5: Food and eating).

Even though Katherine was giving insulin she still developed ketones. This may sound surprising, but some people can become ketotic very quickly, while for others giving regular insulin, even in not the correct amounts, should hold the ketones at bay.

Case 3

Moving from childhood to adulthood

Introducing Jason, 27, diagnosed aged 7

When I was in my early teens I developed fears of my diabetes and I was less open to trying new things. I started using my diabetes as an excuse not to do things, even just leaving the house on my own. I realised there was no one else responsible for me. Suddenly I was in control but I realised that things would happen that I couldn't control.

I drank like anyone else. My hypo symptoms were strong enough to know the difference. I just made sure I ate something after I'd been drinking. I've never been drunk and low. I never smoked or did drugs as I knew it interfered with diabetes.

I was diagnosed when I was 7 and I was in the paediatric clinic until I was 18, then I moved to the adult one. When I was in the kids' clinic I was surrounded by children and there were paintings on the walls by 7-year-olds but it was good – I was encouraged to do sports. I thought, maybe I'm a bit old for this! They left it up to me when to move to the adult clinic. I thought I should go but I didn't like it because it was full of old people – it was more like an OAP clinic and the doctors and nurses weren't as warm and friendly.

I always thought that they [doctors and nurses] didn't understand

Case 3 *continued*

my diabetes as well as I did, and they reinforced it with their knowledge. You can tell clearly if someone has read something in a book and given a textbook answer. It didn't work out and I was transferred to the clinic in my GP practice but GPs are especially governed by structure, keeping to one insulin and not changing it much or your life working around that, living a repetitive life. It would be annoying, they'd say things you've known for years like, 'You can take more insulin if you eat bigger meals', which displays no apparent knowledge.

Last year I asked to be moved to an adult clinic in a hospital and fair dues to them, they really know what they're talking about and they explain things better. Maybe because I was not open before whereas now I'm older and willing to discuss things. Now I don't think I know more than they do.

Discussion

Going through adolescence can be daunting. Jason describes the feeling of being a child and seeing what the adult world holds. Many teenagers want complete independence and control but when Jason caught a glimpse of what it meant in terms of his diabetes, it was a bit daunting. His parents were supporting his care and then when he started being more independent he realised he was in control and things could go wrong. Many, but not all, teenagers are not in this position and they will try and push their personal boundaries and limits – both of the people around them and of their own bodies. Jason was independent from soon after diagnosis at 7 years of age in terms of doing his own injections and blood tests. When making the transition to adulthood, he became very aware of himself and his own limitations. He used his diabetes as an excuse not to smoke or take drugs, a common theme amongst many young people I have spoken to. Peer pressure and the desire to fit in and be the same as one's peers, is a powerful persuader to do everything from working hard to bunking off school, having sex or making a fashion statement.

Jason's experience of the transition process in the hospital clinic sounds like a very lonely one. Being a teenager can be like that – after all, you feel that no one understands you anyway, except perhaps people your own age. If you have diabetes, you may feel incredibly alone. Imagine going to a clinic as a teenager with diabetes – you may think that no one understands you and the doctors are old and crusty and have probably never had sex or drunk alcohol anyway. Even if they have, why would a teenager want to discuss these issues with their diabetes team? It can feel isolating being sat next to a 7-year-old in the outpatients clinic, and depressing sitting next to a 60-year-old in a wheelchair in an adult clinic, wondering if that is what they are going to become in 40 years' time.

Case 4

Leaving the paediatric clinic

Introducing Flin, 23, diagnosed aged 9

I struggled to find a doctor I could relate to as a child and felt really patronised, until I met a doctor when I was 16. I was given a lot of leeway. In the children's clinic there was a rule that once you'd turned 17 your next appointment should be in the adult clinic. I was lucky as I met a doctor 6 months before moving to adult clinic who allowed me to stay until I was 18. It made such a difference. I got on really well with him and we had a mutual respect. I felt I was saying things and he was listening. He was different from the other doctors, who used to have one rule for everybody. We'd talk for 25 minutes about football and then about diabetes. Every time I saw him he knew me. I didn't always have to explain myself. I was able to chat comfortably. Even so, when I was in clinic I never had any education regarding alcohol. I would have been open to it but it never came up and I never brought it up as I felt I shouldn't have been doing it anyway. I was taught it was naughty to have a chocolate and if you eat it you'll be punished with a high blood sugar. I see it the same way with alcohol.

I don't feel my diabetes care has ever been the same since. Now I'm seen in the adult clinic. They don't look at you, they just read off a sheet. I feel that I don't even need to be there, it's just generic care

Case 4 *continued*

and all I am is a number. They're not looking at you and what you need; it's the same rule for everybody. I spend the first half of the appointment just catching up with my treatment over the last five years. There's no consistent doctor – I see a different one each time. You have to come on four separate days to see different health professionals so sometimes you end up missing an appointment.

Discussion

Doctors, nurses and dietitians as well as parents can get out of touch with the needs of young people. Just because a young person does not seem old enough or mature enough to be drinking alcohol or having sex, that doesn't mean they are not doing it. Even if they could be physically prevented from doing these things it would only be a temporary measure.

Moving from the children's to the adults' clinic can feel like a massive shock. Your child will go from seeing the same doctor most of their diabetic life and surrounded by children to sometimes seeing different doctors in a clinic which spans all adult ages. However, there is also a positive spin to growing up – a move away from the screaming kids and into the world of grown-ups. A children's clinic is clearly the wrong setting for a teenager and more hospitals now offer clinics solely for teenagers with more flexibility as to when to transfer care over to the adult team. Many hospitals also run Transition Clinics that combine both paediatric and adult teams. Ideally, it should be the young person's decision as to when they transfer to the adult clinic. However, even in the teenage clinic the real issues that may impact on a young person may not come up, sometimes because priorities in a limited time might be the HbA_{1c}, upcoming exams and getting a driving licence. Or it may be the false belief that the young person sitting in clinic isn't trying sex, alcohol, drugs and cigarettes for themselves.

The teenage years are a particularly important time for young people to form their identity, which carries them through to adult life. During this time it is important that their individual needs are met. Flin struggled to find someone in the medical team he could relate to, and when he did, he was forced to move into adult services. Even when he did, discussions around issues that might impact his diabetes – alcohol, smoking and drugs – did not happen. He tried and experimented with all of them, with no medical guidance. As a parent the best you can do is give your teenager the space to ask questions and gain information, while respecting their privacy. Most teenagers wouldn't be keen to bring up the issue of safe sex with their parents present. This and other topics are relevant to diabetic health (see Chapter 10: Life beyond home). Whilst some responsibility must lie with diabetes teams to broach issues specific to teenagers, some teenagers don't want to talk about these things with their diabetes team. They may feel embarrassed to talk with someone who has known their parents over the years or who has looked after them since childhood, or they may be embarrassed at you being present in clinic. In this case, Flin felt that drinking alcohol was not something he should be doing and any effect it had meant a punishment that he deserved. This may explain why he did not want to bring up the subject in clinic.

Some ideas about how to give young people information about these issues can be found at the end of the chapter, in the section **What you can do**.

Case 5

The important role of the diabetes specialist nurse

Introducing Juliet, 22, diagnosed aged 17

I was diagnosed when I was 17, so I had a year at the children's clinic. I had a really nice nurse who came to my house to visit and I enjoyed going to the children's section of the hospital, it was colourful and friendly. I was quite worrried about moving to adult clinic because that meant changing my nurse. My first nurse in the adult clinic did not offer me as much support as my previous one; he was very busy and would never have the time to come to my house. Trying to ring him was a bit of a nightmare, it was very hard to contact him. And I didn't get on with him as well as my older nurse, who was a warm and friendly person. I could chit-chat to her about lots of other stuff, not just my diabetes, so we were able to build up a relationship. With the other nurse, he just meant business; I had a question about my diabetes, he answered it.

Case 5 *continued*

I changed my nurse soon after and have built up a relationship with her, so when I have my clinic we have a nice chat and talking about my diabetes is just another conversation. She is there for me 100%. If I ring her and she's not around she will always call me back. She's very clued up, but extremely down to earth, which is great. When I see her I don't worry but when I see the doctor I get a bit scared because he has told me off a few times. In my experience doctors are impersonal and they don't know what it 'feels' like to have diabetes, they are just concerned with the HbA$_{1c}$ figures in front of them, and they don't seem to have any empathy towards how it is to live with diabetes on an everyday scale.

Discussion

Moving from the children's to the adult's clinic can be a bit of a culture shock. Juliet was fortunate that she had a nurse in the children's clinic who was able to visit her at home. This is not possible in many clinics that are understaffed.

For Juliet as well as for Flin, building up a relationship with their diabetes team is crucial, so they are known as Flin or Juliet first rather than as Flin or Juliet 'the diabetic'. Some health professionals may not understand this but for young people with diabetes, diabetes is just something that needs to be done and should fit in with their life. Just focusing on diabetes does not allow for a true understanding of how diabetes can impact on a young person's life and how the real dilemmas become intertwined, such as with boyfriends and girlfriends, sport and alcohol. Living with diabetes is very different from managing it in clinic.

There are always going to be 'good' and 'bad' doctors and nurses, but it is worth remembering that there are some who appear antisocial but who may be very good at their jobs and worth listening to. Doctors who run diabetes clinics are usually extremely dedicated. You build up a relationship which is very different from the usual patient–doctor relationship as you get to know each other over many years. The doctors like to think that their patients love them all the time, and while with diabetes you will get very fond of each other over the years there are times when the relationship is strained.

Q Alice is worried about telling her boyfriend she has diabetes. I know it's her decision but I'd feel happier if he and his parents knew in case she has a hypo when they are out together. How can I encourage her to talk more openly about her diabetes with him?

A In this situation if you spill the beans it might never be forgotten or forgiven. However, you also need your daughter to be safe. The first thing you need to do is consider why she doesn't want to tell her boyfriend she has diabetes. She may fear rejection or unneccessary questions, or not want to look different, or it may be part of denying her diabetes to herself. Perhaps she had a previous bad experience and doesn't want to risk it again. Perhaps she is right, why is it necessary to tell all? After all, it is just one thing about Alice. Like all teenagers, Alice will need eventually to take full responsibility for her diabetes, including recognising and treating hypos and making food choices. If she is old enough to choose a boyfriend she is probably old enough to take the responsibility for much of her diabetes care.

What's the worst that will happen? Probably a major hypo or a missed injection, both of which will make Alice feel under the weather. This may blow her cover and cause embarrassment and scare her boyfriend, so it might be worth trying to talk through the possibility of such a scenario before it happens.

In the beginning it was a confidence thing. I didn't want to tell my girlfriend I had diabetes, I didn't want to look different. One day we decided to tell each other things about ourselves for four minutes each. She told me about her sisters. I told her I had diabetes. Before, I was always out with her and she didn't know I had diabetes so I didn't take insulin. The day I did explain she was really interested.

(Daniel, 17)

I had a boyfriend at university. When I told him about my diabetes his parents told him I'd get all these illnesses and he couldn't cope with it. I thought no one would.

(Ruth, 38, who is happily married)

When I was at school I found that it gave people something to be interested in. Boys often think it's quite cool that you can give yourself an injection! It's all about how you sell it in school.

(Nicola, 30)

Q Mark is 18 and has started to go out drinking with friends. I'm worried he may have a hypo and no one will be there to look after him, or even be arrested if police think he is drunk. How can I stop him running into difficulties?

A An active social life can be a barrier to good control. Being a teenager is about exploring and experimenting, which means pushing personal boundaries which may mean taking risks by experimenting with alcohol, sex, drugs, cigarettes or just staying out late. Drinking, smoking, being thin, eating junk food, staying out until the early hours and then sleeping until after lunch are all 'anti-diabetic' and not the recommended routine healthy lifestyle needed for good blood glucose control.

Remember when you were a teenager? What were your main priorities? Probably boyfriends and girlfriends, football, friendships and appearance. Of course everyone is different: some teenagers are very focused on work, music and sport. If this is the case, management of their diabetes will be a focus, as having hypos during a football match or orchestra practice isn't ideal. If it isn't, they may want to forget they have diabetes completely. This is a bit like covering your eyes and saying 'You can't see me!'

Some people may 'super-normalise' themselves, to prove how normal they are, which may mean pushing the boundaries even

continued on next page

A *continued*

further. Sometimes it is just up to the individual to realise when they have reached their own limits. It will be hard for you to stand by and let this happen without going on about their diabetes, which may make your teenager want to cover up what they are doing even more.

If you want to minimise risks it is best that you allow your teenager to be informed. This is true for those without diabetes as well, when it comes to teenage issues like unprotected sex, taking drugs, partying late, alcohol and smoking; but if you have diabetes, the need is more pressing as they can all interfere with blood glucose control. Chances are you won't know how to advise your teenager on their diabetic care when it comes to these issues. It'll be no use telling them they can't leave the house – this won't be sustainable for very long or you may find them climbing out of their bedroom window! You will need to create an opportunity for your teenager to talk through these things with someone they respect, and this may not be anyone in their diabetes team. Young persons' groups are good places to give and share information, so ask the diabetes team if they run or know of such groups. The internet also has some useful resources for teenagers with diabetes (see the Appendix). If your teenager still goes to the children's clinic, the team there may not be in the habit of thinking about 'adult' issues. If you bring this up with the team, they may offer to have a conversation with your teenager, but this is likely only if you are not in the room. It may be time for you to come to terms with the fact that you do not have complete control over your child's life. Given that you have looked after them from a baby, this can feel terrifying.

Friends tell me not to smoke but they do too so they don't have a leg to stand on. I like smoking. Even if it makes you die earlier I'll carry on. If I drink, I'll be low at lunchtime the next day and eat an extra bag of crisps. People say things like, don't you have to inject when you're drinking, or, I thought you weren't allowed to drink if you're diabetic.

(Luke, 17)

I started going to pubs when I was about 16.
I went into three [hypoglycaemic] diabetic comas
related to alcohol. It was a wake-up call.
After that I'd give less insulin and eat more
food if I'd been out drinking. I never wanted
to smoke. Diabetes gave me an excuse not to
give in to peer pressure. It was useful. I'd
say, 'I can't smoke, I'll lose a leg'. Friends
would stop offering. When I tried cannabis and
speed I wasn't thinking about my diabetes.

(Katherine, 30)

When I was in my early teens my pastimes were
football. I kept my head down. I was in the top sets at
school. When I was 15 I started drinking alcohol. I was
looking for other things to entertain myself with and to
push the boundaries. My diabetes was pushed futher down
my list of priorities. If I was told not to do something
I would have turned around and done it. I used to
experiment with draw [cannabis]. You don't know what
you're feeling, you lose all control. The last thing you'll do
is a blood test. Once I was completely out of it. I had
to admit to my Mum that I had been smoking draw. She
was relieved as I wasn't having a hypo. I realised I had
overdone it, it was a wake-up call. I realised that it had
an impact on my health and my diabetes because I lost
control. Being in control of my diabetes had always been
a big thing. After that I used my diabetes as an excuse
with friends. I'd say, 'My sugars haven't been good today'.
Now I know I have my limits.

(Flin, 23)

I always carry a blood testing machine with me. Once
you've done a blood test when you're drinking a couple
of times you know what happens to your body and so
you know what to do.

(Nigel, 37)

In the morning I'll be high after drinking and then by mid-morning I'll be low. I tend to stick to the same drinks, but that's advisable for all of us.

(Mike, 27)

When I used to go out drinking I'd wake up with a headache. I didn't know if it was a hangover or a hypo. I learnt that I'd drop by mid-morning so I had to eat something before I go to bed.

(Lucia, 37)

Q Ella doesn't seem the slightest bit interested in her diabetes. She's out with her friends and sometimes I find her long-acting insulin left in her bedroom. I feel like a constant nag. How can I get her more interested in her diabetes?

A At 15, Ella may not be interested in seeing beyond the next few days or weeks, whereas your priority may be for her to have good control to avoid complications in the next 10, 20 or 30 years and beyond. This tug-of-war between what you as a parent want and what Ella wants may cause you anxiety and distress. You may feel like locking her up and carrying on treating her as a child, as you may feel that is how she is acting anyway. Remember back to when you were a teenager; what you wanted was to hang out with your friends and fit in. Fitting in may involve drinking, smoking, doing drugs and having sex.

Ella's lack of self-care may involve several factors. She may be trying to pretend to herself and her friends that she doesn't have diabetes. Missing injections and partying all night and surviving it may be evidence for that. She may also be angry she has diabetes and is just beginning to realise that it will last forever. Perhaps she is deliberately missing injections to control her weight (see Chapter 5: Food and eating). At some point you are going to have to let go

continued

completely, but maybe not yet. Let go but always be there to see how it's been, and be willing to take back control as and when she will let you.

Learning how to adapt to drinking alcohol will help teenagers avoid hypos. However, they may not want to discuss issues like alcohol, sex and smoking with their parents, so you will need to allow them the opportunity to do so when you aren't there, otherwise these important topics may never come up.

It is important to try and ease the teenage years as much as possible to optimise blood glucose control and minimise the risk of complications. Poor control in the teenage years can set the foundation for complications in the future and at its extreme can interfere with nomal growth. Teenagers still like parents to set boundaries, just as children do. It shows them that you care, even if it causes doors to slam. At the end of the day, your teenager is going to have to live with their diabetes and incorporate it in their life. You will have to let them make some mistakes.

I didn't used to get around to doing my blood tests. Now I test 4–5 times in a week. It benefits me a lot more. I have a confidence thing about my weight and height. Friends tower above me. I'm still trying to get there. I don't want to feel small. If my diabetes was better controlled I could get bigger. I'm trying to be more normal in my physical appearance.

(Daniel, 17)

When I was a teenager I could go a couple of days without doing a blood test. Mum used to be on my case so I wouldn't do a test.

(Flin, 23)

I never wanted to let diabetes stop me enjoying myself.

(Jane, 34)

I don't care about diabetes. I only care about what I'm going to do when I'm old. I want to live by myself.

(Kiet, 16)

I make excuses, like today it's because I've been busy. I don't have much foresight. I look to tomorrow, not the future. I test every so often.

(Luke, 17)

Mum still does some injections for me when I can't be bothered.

(Summer, 13)

Q **The doctor in the clinic has suggested that Nick is seen on his own. I don't feel happy about this. At the end of the day it's me that has to pick up the pieces. Are the doctors right or should I push to stay in control?**

A It's time for you to back off a little. If Nick (15) is keen to be seen on his own then you should allow it. If he is monosyllabic about the idea it doesn't mean he isn't interested, he may just be thinking about it. Perhaps you could suggest coming in at the end of the consultation. It will be important that Nick is allowed the opportunity to talk through things he may find he doesn't want to talk about with you there, such as alcohol and staying out late. You will need to respect the fact that he speaks to his diabetes team in private and not expect the team or him to tell you what has been discussed, or he may never want to see them again. It could be a golden opportunity for Nick to start feeling the responsibilities of living an adult life with his diabetes.

I don't like Mum being there. If I say things in front of her she gives me a dodgy look. Some things you don't know how to say.

(Summer, 13)

In adult clinic I saw a different doctor every time. They didn't know me on a personal basis, they just saw me as a number. They saw a diabetic teenager not looking after themselves. Actually I needed deep emotional help, not telling me I would die.

(Martina, 28)

When I was diagnosed, mum was hysterical. There was a time when she wanted to get very involved, reminding me all the time. But a diabetes nurse who was visiting me at home told mum to let me deal with it. It's better now, it got mum off my back.

(Luke, 17)

I stayed in kids' clinic till I was 18. When I changed it was like suddenly there was me and everyone else in their 60s.

(James, 28)

Q Fiona wants to apply for a driving licence. The DVLA form asks for her doctor's details, to contact about Fiona's diabetes. We have discussed driving with her doctor, but the doctor says Fiona's blood glucose is not stable enough. Is this discrimination?

A You and Fiona may feel she is being discriminated against by having her doctor contacted by DVLA. It is annoying and it is a direct result of having diabetes, which was uninvited and unwanted in the first place, and this may well make you both feel angry. However, at the end of the day if Fiona's blood glucose levels are unstable out of a car, they may also be unstable behind the wheel of a car. Getting

continued on next page

continued

behind a wheel is pretty dangerous anyway. Having a hypo on the road can kill not only the person behind the wheel but also other drivers, cyclists and pedestrians. It may be the perfect motivator for Fiona to improve her blood glucose levels. It is up to her to convince her doctor that she has a sensible and knowledgeable attitude to driving.

It is important to do a blood test before driving, if feeling tired or funny whilst driving and always to have enough food readily available to treat a hypo. A big hypo whilst driving may result in the licence being taken away and even being charged and prosecuted.

It's a pain to have to renew your driving licence every 3 years but it's one of those things that has to be accepted. I don't see it as discrimination, it's just a pain. These things have to be done; it's not just your safety it's everybody else's.

(Flin, 23)

I've had no problems driving, just a few hypos but I've turned off the road when I realised and I have quite good warning symptoms. I pretty much always test before getting in the car now.

(Jane, 34)

Often I drive long distances. Sometimes I'm driving and I think I'm a bit tired and I think it's just driving fatigue but when I get to my destination my blood might be low or high. It's just a funny sensation. Driving fatigue can cloud your judgement. Now I always test before driving long distances and if I feel funny en route. I always have some Dextrose [glucose tablets] and snack bars with me.

(Flin, 23)

I've never had a hypo when driving. I always keep Dextrose and a cereal bar in the car just in case though. On long journeys I do a blood test before I set off.
I find it a hassle updating my driving licence every 3 years. On the plus side I got to update the terrible photograph on my driving licence for free, rather than having to wait until I'm 70.

(Nicola, 30)

What you can do

- **Be ready to give up responsibilities** but also be prepared to supervise and take some responsibility back if needed.

- **Let your teenager make a few mistakes** while you watch in the wings and make sure no major events occur. The odd high blood glucose level because of a delayed injection is not serious, but if this occurs regularly it can be. It's important that a teenager is allowed to experiment a bit, as this is crucial to setting their own boundaries and eventually their own set of rules by which they are to live.

- **Talk through some possible scenarios before they happen.** For example, who would they like to tell they have diabetes – one new friend or a teacher at school or their new girlfriend? Think what will happen if there is a hypo or hyper and no one knows; how would they like to deal with it? If no one knows and they are out and about and need an injection, what could they do?

- **Allow the opportunity** for your teenager to talk through things that they may not want to discuss with you, such as sex, cigarettes, alcohol and drugs. It is much better to do this before opportunities arise and they impulsively think, Why not? It may mean you do not come to their hospital appointments, or agree only to come in at the end of the appointment. Your teenager may not want to talk either to you or their doctor about such issues but providing information is important so they have knowledge and know where to look for it. There are also teenage internet websites that talk about these issues (see the Appendix). The specialist nurse in the clinic may know some good websites, or if you find one you could write it on a piece of paper and leave it on your child's desk. Curiosity may make them look at it in their own time.

- **Encourage your child to be into something** that requires some discipline, such as music, sport or a hobby. Having an interest in something, anything, that they enjoy may help provide a motivation for improving blood gucose control and a distraction from focusing solely on diabetes.
- The bottom line is, **talk about it!**

Rachel's view

I never had a major teenage rebellion, my rebellion came a little later. All of us have one, although some are shorter than others. As a teenager I was into work and sport, and I started getting interested in amateur dramatics. Having a hypo on stage would have been a real no-no and I would have forgotten my lines so I had the motivation to stay on track.

Sometimes when my bloods misbehaved I would get annoyed, mostly at myself. I was the quiet teenager who seemed quite content but on the inside I was fuming. This has driven me over the years to achieve a lot but it's been a tiring task. As I reached my late teens and I started going to parties and drinking alcohol, I found my bloods a bit more erratic but not massively so. Doing exams really sent my bloods up the spout. I wouldn't change my insulin dose but they would be quite high before an exam. If I corrected them I would have a big hypo during the exam as I settled into it and the adrenaline rush wore off. If I didn't correct them, my blood would be fine when I came out. A few days before a big exam I would try and eat the same breakfast and work out how much insulin my body needed exactly, to get through the exam without thinking about my bloods and making sure they were spot on so I could perform.

My diabetes was always well-controlled when at home as many life stresses were taken care of for me by my parents, such as cooking meals and not worrying about income. It allowed me to do my thing and think about my diabetes. Having stability at home, a routine and good diabetes control has set me up for life. Children who don't have this stability at home are at a massive disadvantage in terms of support and optimal blood glucose control, which may creep up on them in the longer term. This injustice is what upsets me the most when I see children and young people with diabetes, who are products of where they come from.

Life beyond home

Are there any jobs you can't do if you have diabetes treated with insulin?

There are some jobs which are banned if you have diabetes treated with insulin. These include the armed forces, certain parts of the transport industry, oil rigs, and so on. Some careers may be restricted if you have diabetes and may be subject to individual assessment. However, working in emergency care, for example as a firefighter, nurse or doctor, is allowed, although an individual must be fit for duty and this will be assessed on an individual basis.

Legislation governing these areas is often reviewed, so seek advice from the careers office or the licensing authority in the area of interest: there are contact details in the Appendix.

Are there any problems with having children if you have diabetes?

Many couples with diabetes have healthy babies but planning when to get pregnant is important. There are risks to the mother and to the developing fetus. Risks can be greatly reduced by optimising blood glucose control before and during pregnancy. For this reason, extremely tight blood glucose control for several months before as well as during pregnancy is important. The risk of neural tube defects is higher in babies born to mothers with diabetes, so it is recommended that women with diabetes take 5 mg folic acid daily before becoming pregnant and during the first 12 weeks of pregnancy. This is a much higher dose than is taken by mothers who do not have diabetes.

There are special clinics for those with diabetes who are pregnant to help achieve as good blood glucose levels as possible and to monitor the expectant mother and baby during the pregnancy. This may include extra ultrasound scans, monitoring of blood glucose levels and assessment of diabetes-related complications. Mothers with diabetes are more likely to have big babies who may have low blood sugars after being born. The baby's blood glucose levels are normally monitored after birth (by doing a simple and quick heel prick blood test before and sometimes after a feed) so they can be treated if they drop. There are some other specific problems, most of which can be prevented with tight blood glucose control in pregnancy. For the mother, there can be damage to vessels in the backs of the eyes and to the kidneys during pregnancy; this will need to be monitored carefully so treatment can be given if needed. Strict recommendations for the care of pregnant women with diabetes have been drawn up by the National Institute of Clinical Excellence (www. nice.org.uk).

There are also diabetic complications which may make conception more difficult. Sometimes men in later life have erectile dysfunction, and women may suffer with loss of libido, losing their interest in sex.

Does having diabetes affect insurance policies?

Getting insurance can be an issue if you have diabetes because of the risk of complications; often premiums are higher than if you don't have diabetes. It is worth shopping around as you may find a big difference in policy and prices between insurance companies. Diabetes UK provides very helpful insurance services: see their website for more information.

Will diabetes affect recreational activities such as parachuting, flying a plane or scuba diving?

Lone parachute jumping is not normally allowed due to risk of hypoglycaemia, although tandem parachute jumps are usually permitted.

In the UK, for diabetes treated by insulin, which will be those with Type 1 diabetes or Type 2 treated with insulin, applicants can apply for a restricted licence to fly a plane. This means that you can only fly solo or with a safety pilot and not carry passengers. There are strict critieria which need to be met which include good diabetes control and good hypoglycaemia awareness, without requiring third party assistance. A doctor will need to countersign a medical declaration saying you are fit to learn to fly through discussion with a Medical Advisor at the Civil Aviation Authority. Any flying instructor will need to be satisfied that you meet the requirements or you will be refused permission to fly. Further information can be found on the Civil Aviation Authority website (www.caa.co.uk).

The main concern with scuba diving is having an unexpected hypo when under water causing loss of consciousness and drowning. Some of the same feelings experienced when hypo may mimic the diving-related 'decompression sickness', otherwise known as 'the bends'. Each needs speedy identification and management but very different treatment. This has caused a great potential anxiety in the scuba diving community as well as an outcry amongst those in the diabetes community who want to scuba dive. Scuba diving in the UK is permitted under rules set out by the UKSDMC (UK Sport Diving Medical Committee), which have been relaxed over the past decade. In practical terms these restrict diving in the UK due to the recommendation that those with diabetes must not have experienced hypoglycaemia within the past year, even though hypoglycaemia, even if mild, is a likely occurrence in all people with diabetes, unless blood glucose control is poor with blood glucose levels persistently running high. Other restrictions include diabetes-related complications. Further information, advice and application forms are found via the website (www.uksdmc.co.uk).

There are differences in restrictions and guidelines abroad, so if you are travelling it would be wise to contact the UKSDMC in advance for advice, and if one exists, a diving association in the country where you will want to scuba dive, in case you need to bring a medical letter with you. It is best to be up front about your diabetes and to follow medical and diving advice.

Further information about international scuba diving can be found at the Divers Alert Network (www. diversalertnetwork.org).

Case 1

Getting the most out of life

Introducing Jason, 27, diagnosed aged 7

Having diabetes has made me more determined. It could hold you back and doesn't make things as simple as everyone else's lives, so you want to prove it to yourself and others that you can do things and that you can do it really well. As a result I have ended up

continued on next page

achieving the most in my family academically and career-wise. I am renowned for being a high achiever.

Having diabetes makes you want to enjoy life. It puts life into perspective as it gives you a sense of mortality. Life is delicate and precious; it could end at any time. You're doing something all the time to keep yourself alive – it makes you a lot more open-minded and wanting to enjoy life. I am lucky to be here; 100 years ago I might not have been around.

Introducing Susie, 24, diagnosed aged 8

I have always pushed myself really hard and had high expectations in all aspects of my life, including my diabetes. I don't know if I would have been like that anyway or whether my diabetes has been a factor. When I was growing up I never wanted my diabetes to stop me doing anything, so it made me do more than I would have done anyway just to prove it to myself. I often wonder what life would have been like if I didn't have diabetes, but I'll never know. That gets me down sometimes but it also makes me more determined.

When I've got a lot on, my diabetes is the first thing that slips because it's there all the time. Sometimes I think about my diabetes a lot and just wish it would go away. At other times it's just one of the jobs I need to do during the day. Other people don't realise because I don't make a fuss about it and that can also be hard because it makes me feel alone sometimes.

There was a time when my diabetes felt too much to cope with. My life was stressful at that time anyway while I was at college and diabetes on top of it felt too much. On my own I would suddenly start crying for no apparent reason. I used to cry myself to sleep most nights. I was still trying hard with my diabetes as best as I could but my HbA_{1c} slipped to around 8.8%, so not a major disaster, but it felt like it for me. I started to not cope. I felt out of control. Doing blood tests was even too much and I stopped doing them. I had always been a bad sleeper but one night I couldn't sleep at all and felt as if I wasn't part of the world and was looking at everyone from

Case 1 *continued*

the outside. I was really scared I might start missing my injections. I waited for my friend outside her house that morning and confessed to her that I wasn't coping and asked her to help me. I hadn't had a hospital appointment for a year because the hospital had forgotten to send me one, although I had tried to make one and had left a couple of messages with the appointment people. Because I was so miserable I couldn't motivate myself to try harder. I felt exhausted by everything but still put on a smile for everyone else except for me. Inside I felt alone, a big failure and not worthwhile. Every high blood test seemed to reinforce that feeling. My diabetes felt like a chain around my neck.

My friend managed to easily organise an appointment for me in the hospital and I did get some support. A lot has happened since then and now I wear my smile from the inside out. I am scared that I could go back to those feelings but I have learnt that I need to look after my mind and my body. I constantly try, but it is hard to balance work, life, food and diabetes. My job is stressful and unpredictable and I want a life, so I try and cut myself a bit of slack and do the best I can. But being a perfectionist I still find it hard when my blood's high, like I'm a big failure. I'll just have to hope that my best is good enough.

Discussion

Depression is higher in those with diabetes than those without. Having diabetes can sometimes feel like too much to cope with, on top of everything else. Although feeling 'down' because of diabetes may seem 'reasonable' as an explanation, it does not mean that the problem should not be addressed. Like Jason as well as Susie in these cases, many people with diabetes strive to achieve their goals, trying to prove to themselves that they can be and that they are in fact 'normal'. Many appear to be 'super-normal', determined to get the most out of life. The flip side is that sometimes this can be a struggle, and with diabetes it is easy to feel isolated. The burden of living with diabetes, on top of trying to achieve and push personal boundaries, can sometimes mean that blood glucose control slips. Diabetes became overwhelming for Susie at one stage in her life. It is difficult to know whether her worsening blood glucose levels were the cause of her feeling a failure or the other way around, perhaps a bit of both. Either way, this loss of self-care can have detrimental effects, although fortunately Susie still retained some insight and was able to seek help. It would be worth considering if your child is starting to lose self-care, whether they are just exploring and experimenting or whether perhaps their mood is the cause. Susie asked for help and received it. How each of us chooses to live our life has to be a personal, but informed decision. As parents, all you can do is carry on loving your children, 'being there' for them and hope they love you back. You will never stop worrying about them.

Case 2

Concerns about travelling

Introducing Juliet, 22, diagnosed aged 17

Travelling is definitely one thing that worries me in terms of my diabetes. It scares me and it would be really nice to talk to someone with diabetes who has gone away to weird and wonderful places. I worry about keeping my insulin cool and about whether I would need to bring a HUUUUGE supply of medication with me. I think it would be a right pain in the bum having to bring six months' supply: you'd need a whole other suitcase! Saying that, however much it worries me, when the time comes for me to travel I won't let it stop me.

My parents would definitely be worried about me and my diabetes if I went travelling. They always say that they want me to go to nice 'Westernised places', when I think they really mean 'We want her to go somewhere where she can look after her diabetes properly'!

Travelling is the only obstacle really that I think I face with my diabetes. I have had many chances to go travelling ... since leaving Uni many of my friends have asked me. Up until now I've said no, but only because I want to work for a few years and save up all my money. At the back of my mind, every time we sit around talking about how fantastic travelling would be I think 'Ahhhhh what would I do about my

Case 2 *continued*

diabetes?' Then I get a bit down. I do feel envious of everybody else who don't have to worry about something like that. If people worry about 'Ooh what clothes would you bring?' and superficial stuff like that I think, 'Shut up! Least you haven't got to worry about your medication!'

Introducing Flin, 23, diagnosed aged 9

I went travelling when I was 19 and I was away for 5 months. Not the best timing, but a month before I set off I changed my insulin. I was travelling with a friend and he took a spare set of everything. Mum had supplies sent to me on my trip and my uncle met me with some more along the way. I was in New York in the snow and Los Angeles which was over hot. I hate having to be on a beach and inject, it's my worst nightmare. I had food poisoning in Sri Lanka, I was being sick all night and the next day I took a five-hour taxi drive. Foods were different and I had to deal with time zones. But it didn't ruin my experience at all. It started to make me do blood tests again.

Introducing Nigel, 37, diagnosed aged 3

After leaving school I went to the Australian Bush for six weeks and hoed cotton with the Aborigines. I had tried to get a job in Sydney but I didn't get one, although that's where my Mum thought I was! I met someone in Sydney who said, 'If you're tough you can do cotton shipping. There are lots of jobs but no one lasts more than a day'. I thought, 'I've got to do it'. I only had fifteen pounds to my name and I was 12,000 miles from home. Mum and Dad couldn't just turn up.

When I arrived, the Aborigines thought I wouldn't be able to hack it. I would get up and start work at 4 a.m. and work until 2 p.m. by which time it was 50 degrees centigrade. The Abos couldn't believe I could do it as a white man, let alone with diabetes. I became a superhero. I had to lower my insulin dramatically as the heat and work had a massive effect.

It was so hot that I had my spare insulin in a thermos flask, but even so it all went cloudy after a few days. To get some more the pharmacy had to parachute me in some more with the weekly 10 a.m. Tuesday morning drop. It landed in a dusty old paddock.

Discussion

Doing anything completely new for the first time, although exciting, can also be a bit scary. I expect Juliet would be excited and apprehensive about travelling anyway. All the 'what ifs' could stop her going, but when you read the gusto in her stories in other chapters it is clear that her diabetes won't stop her. Juliet was diagnosed a year before leaving home and is less well rehearsed at living with diabetes than Flin or Nigel. At diagnosis she relied on her parents for support and for some of the practical issues relating to diabetes. She is starting to get a bit cross with her parents treating her in the same way as when she was diagnosed. Of course this is not her parents' fault. They haven't changed, she has. She is gaining confidence in her diabetes as she gets older. So with this change her parents will need to try and be less anxious and let her experiment. She'll do it anyway, with or without her parents worrying. Juliet and her parents could do with talking to someone with diabetes who has travelled successfully, like Flin or Nigel, then she can start planning her big trip with fewer anxieties all round.

Flin and Nigel were both experienced with their diabetes before travelling, however they still had to learn by their mistakes, and this was part of their emergence into adult life. The process of travelling helped Flin to decide about the need to do blood tests, think for himself and plan ahead. Some things just can't be anticipated, like illnesses abroad, but Flin was able to get around this. Nothing was impossible. He would do things differently next time but it didn't ruin his experience. Similarly for Nigel, he thought he had anticipated the heat but his insulin still went off; nevertheless, he was able to organise a new supply even in the remote Australian Bush.

Case 3

Going to college
Introducing Nicola, 30, diagnosed aged 11

I went to university when I was 18. I found the first year quite difficult, mainly because I left behind a close family, really good friends and the security of home. Diabetes was just another thing to cope with.

Case 3 *continued*

My parents had always supported me in getting prescriptions, looking after me when I was hypo, and just general moral support, and taking complete responsibility for myself felt like hard work and was quite scary at times. It is preparation for real life though. I got through it by telling the close friends I'd made about the ins and outs of diabetes, and what to do if I said I was hypo. That made me feel less alone. I soon got into the swing of remembering to update prescriptions. It's just about getting used to the responsibility.

Before I went to university my doctor gave me some great advice. He said that there would be lots of temptations at university. He said that if I lived a wild life for 3 years, so long as I did my best with my diabetes, it wouldn't have a dramatic effect on my health, so just have fun! I did do my best with my diabetes, but inevitably when there is so much else going on it's not that easy to maintain great control. The doctor's advice meant that I relaxed about it, and did really enjoy myself. He was right, too. Once I had left university and settled down into a 9–5 lifestyle my diabetes became much easier to control.

One thing that I learned about was my long-acting insulin. I used to wonder why on really late nights out I would get so much more tired than my friends. Then I realised that I usually took my long-acting insulin at 'bed time' which could be any time between 10 p.m. and 4 a.m. This would mean that on a late night out I could be up to six hours late with my insulin, and hence be feeling quite groggy. Of course this wasn't helped by alcohol, the need for sleep and the chips on the way home.

Introducing Juliet, 22, diagnosed aged 17

Uni was great. I made so many friends, studied and played hard and diabetes did not get in the way once. All my friends were very supportive and always made sure I was OK. It was like they took the place of my parents while I was at Uni.

When I went to Uni I had only had diabetes for a year. I was really scared about Freshers week – two weeks of constant drinking and late nights. I didn't know how I was going to manage that with my diabetes; would I be able to get my trusty 'diet coke and vodka' that I always drank to help maintain my blood sugars on a night out?

However, Freshers week was the funniest two weeks of my life. I looked after myself, checked my sugars regularly, and made sure I drank my trusty diet coke. I was able to get involved in all the drinking games, I just didn't drink the cheap Lambrini and beer that everybody else did. That definitely saved my waistline a little bit.

There would be some nights throughout Uni where I thought 'bugger it' and tried to drink like everybody else, but that was a very silly mistake. My sugars would be very, very high and I would end up giving myself a jab of insulin. Then I'd find myself going hypo a little while later. Because of my diabetes I never got as drunk or out of control as a lot of people did. I find this a little blessing in disguise. I did have a few times when I got too drunk, but I was OK, although I did suffer the next day. Apart from feeling crap, my sugars were very hard to control.

The constant going out drinking did catch up on me and I experienced the effects at both ends of the scale. I would often walk around campus with a Lucozade bottle in my hand because my sugars would be very low the next day. Other times if I ate something very fatty when I got in at, say, 3 a.m., then I would wake up and have extremely high sugars and feel crap. After my first year at Uni my HbA$_{1c}$ gradually got worse and I knew I had to sort it out. Consequently, my second and third year weren't so crazy on the drinking front, but they were just as fun and I felt a lot better in myself.

After 3 years of lots of drinking, partying and late nights I'm pretty much an expert in terms of my diabetes and alcohol. I know exactly what I can and can't handle, and how to deal with it.

Sometimes I do get down about having to be extra careful. Sometimes when I'm out it seems that everyone has no worries, no cares and I have to go to the loo and do my insulin again. And sometimes my sugars are low and I have to take some time out and eat my Dextrose tablets or my sugars are high and I have to deliberate whether or not to do a little injection, and if I don't I do spend some of my night worrying and thinking 'Ahhhh my sugars are really high right now' and I hate that.

Coping with exams at Uni wasn't too difficult and never bothered me. I get quite nervous before my exam and I always think 'Ahhhhhh I think I'm hypo', but I'm not, it's just the adrenaline pumping about which feels like a hypo. The examiners were very supportive about my diabetes. Before going into the exam hall I'd just tell them I had diabetes and that I had my blood kit and sugar tablets with me.

Introducing Flin, 23, diagnosed aged 9

I've always been independent and had been brought up cooking and ironing my own clothes. There was so much more I was apprehensive about in going to Uni, not related to diabetes. Unfortunately I went 3 years while I was at Uni without seeing a specialist. I was supposed to be referred after leaving the children's clinic but these things take time, and if you don't push, it doesn't happen. I was doing sport seven days a week, socialising, eating and drinking a lot. During that time, having come back from travelling, I started to test my bloods more, whereas as a teenager I could go a couple of days without doing a blood test, not out of protest but because I felt I didn't need to. Now I couldn't do that. Going to Uni and travelling I became more conscious of it. Now I'll do a quick test just to see how I am.

My worst thing is missing my Lantus [once-a-day long-acting insulin] when I haven't gone home when I normally would, so I catch up the next day with half the amount and some short-acting insulin. I don't know if that's the right thing to do, but that's what I do. Sometimes I'm absolutely fine, other times it doesn't matter how much insulin I take, my bloods are still high.

Discussion

You may be horrified to read these stories about drinking, staying out late and partying. You may want to try to persuade your children when they leave home to be 'sensible'.

If your child wants to go on to further education and move away from home it can be frightening both for you and them. You will need to let your child go. You will have to accept you will no longer have the same level of control; you will not know that they have eaten or given their injection. It's time to trust them. This time is an extension of the teenage years and time for your child to use the skills they have learnt to manage on their own. However, the environment will be new and the temptations and influences diverse, so the experimenting will not stop yet. Doing everything for yourself away from home can be a lot to take on anyway. It's their time for a new beginning and most rise splendidly to this challenge. A few stumbles on the way never hurt anyone, and can be a lot of fun too.

Letting go completely will be hard. Doing it in steps as your children grow up will help both you and them.

Nicola and Juliet both decided to share their diabetes with their new friends. It was the right decision for them and allowed them to grow in their self-confidence as well as reducing their feeling of being a bit different because of their diabetes.

Learning by mistakes is important because it allows a young person to set their own rules and decide how they want to live in adult life. You can't always protect your children from everything, much as you'd like to.

Juliet learnt that she felt better when her blood glucose levels were more stable and that was her motivation to look after herself. Juliet is her own expert and knows what works for her. Despite trial and error she has had no disasters and feels proud of herself and in control.

Flin also learnt from his experiences and there was a positive effect in that he decided to start doing blood tests more regularly again. He found something that sort of works for him if he stays out and misses his long-acting insulin. He hasn't brought this up with his diabetes team. Just like with drinking, it's because he feels he is 'naughty' and shouldn't be doing it, even though everyone else around him is (see Chapter 9: The teenage years).

Some responsibility must lie with diabetes clinics to tackle these issues. It would also help to stop making young people feel guilty. Why shouldn't Flin go out until late? If someone could troubleshoot how to get around these issues his blood glucose and quality of life would improve, I expect mostly from being permitted to behave like any other young person his age without the guilt.

There is often conflict between leading a 'good diabetic life' and a feeling of wanting to be free. Being free for some may mean ignoring diabetes. There is a balance to be struck and this is a personal choice. During times of new exploration the balance may fall to new adventure with diabetes taking a back seat. Hopefully the pendulum swings back to a comfortable middle ground with good diabetes control and a good quality of life.

Chances are you will be the one at home worrying whilst your children are out having fun. Maybe it's time to pamper yourself and enjoy the extra time you have, rather than replace it with more worrying. Your children will no doubt come back with a pile of dirty washing and to raid your fridge and cupboards. They will know that you are there for them if and when they need you. That is usually enough.

Case 4

Relationships

Introducing Melanie, 27, diagnosed aged 15

When it comes to being careful about sex I border on the obsessive because of the requirement to control your blood sugars before conception and during pregnancy. I think it has influenced the way I am when I come to sleeping with people. I make sure and take precautions – I use double contraception! It's difficult not to consider the risk of getting pregnant each time you have sex and totally relax about the whole thing. Your body's going 'Come on!' and your mind's going 'Hold on!' If I gave birth to a baby with problems because I hadn't controlled my blood sugars I couldn't cope with the guilt. I don't know if I'd be able to live with myself. Often I do everything but intercourse and I still worry for a split second: what if I get pregnant? You can worry about pregnancy so much that your mind plays tricks on you.

If I'm on a date, over dinner I'll pull out my injection and say 'Do you mind if I do my injection – I'm diabetic'. I don't think much about it. Here's me, take it or leave it. Boyfriends ask me lots of questions. I paint a matter-of-fact picture about my diabetes.

Once I was snogging this guy and I hadn't had my evening Lantus

continued on next page

Case 4 *continued*

[long-acting insulin]. It was four in the morning, my mouth was all dry and I was worrying about what he was thinking. He must have thought, 'I'm snogging a biscuit!'

Once a boyfriend's brother said 'God made you diabetic and theoretically you should be dead'. I turned around and said 'Well if that's the case then God wouldn't have discovered insulin then would he.'

Every now and then you still come across someone who is totally ignorant and doesn't know anything about diabetes. They say things like, 'You can't eat chocolate'. That's the main one. 'You must be used to your injections by now' is the other one.

Introducing George, 35, diagnosed aged 9
Between the ages of 12 and 17 I developed thrush on my penis. I was too embarrassed to say anything about it. I didn't realise that is was due to my high blood sugars. It put me off sex. I lack confidence because of my diabetes. Every girl wants a bloke to be perfect.

Discussion

Melanie is clearly aware of the risks of having an unplanned pregnancy with diabetes. It has influenced how she is in sexual relationships because of her worries, even though she is aware that she is a bit overanxious. In some ways this may be a good thing, at least there will be no mistakes! However, the guilt that goes hand in hand with diabetes can reduce people's enjoyment of the pleasures in life. Many people with diabetes become very good planners and organisers, and that is necessary. Many also have talked to me about being in control of their blood glucose levels, their bodies, their food, their alcohol. Melanie is also in control when it comes to sex. Is this a bad thing? I suppose only if it is a worry for her. It was difficult to find men to talk to me about sex and if there is a worry in relation to their diabetes. Most did not own up to worries over potential impotence with poor blood glucose control. It is difficult to see how something that is working could stop some time, even if you are told that it may. This is true for all diabetic complications (see Chapter 6: Hyperglycaemia, ketoacidosis and complications).

George has had a negative experience when he was younger relating to thrush on his penis because of high blood glucose levels. He didn't feel able to bring up such a personal issue to his diabetes team and they didn't know to ask him.

Q Ella wants to go travelling for several months before she starts university. Is it safe?

A As long as Ella is well prepared then it shouldn't be a problem. A lot needs to be organised before heading off and diabetes also needs thinking about. If someone does want to go travelling, they usually do not want to end up in hospital but want to enjoy their experience. This is often enough motivation to get blood glucose levels in enough check to be safe when travelling. It makes travelling easier if you can go with someone else, because they can carry spares of everything you need in case things get lost or stolen, and if there are any problems they can contact someone else. However, travelling alone is possible, even if a bit daunting to some. There's a lot to think about and something is bound not to have been anticipated, which is in part why people go travelling in the first place, to have new experiences.

However, there are some things which can be thought about in advance.

- Get double the supplies you need, and store half in a separate bag in case one bag gets lost or stolen.
- When crossing time zones, advance planning can make the change go relatively smoothly, and if not smoothly it will sort itself out pretty quickly if enough blood tests are done and they are acted upon. Discuss any need to change insulin dose or timing with the diabetes team before setting off.
- New food can be a challenge, but again this is part of the travelling experience, but it does mean a willingness to do extra blood tests and correct high blood glucose levels if needed.
- Keep insulin supplies in your hand luggage when flying, to avoid the low temperatures in the luggage hold.

continued on next page

A *continued*

- Carry a letter, and a copy, in case of problems through security checks.
- Think of the worst case scenario, like losing all your insulin or blood testing kit and work out the solutions in advance. Find out if there is a diabetes organisation in the country you are visiting, as well as where you could buy extra insulin, and what type would be available. Specific insulin manufacturers (see Appendix) will be able to tell you if your insulin is available locally if needs be.
- Make sure diabetes is covered on your travel and health insurance.
- Your diabetes team will be able to give specific advice about taking supplies, how your insulin and testing kit is affected by different climates, what to do if things go wrong and time zones.

I've been away by myself a few times on sailing and windsurfing holidays in Turkey and Greece. Travelling abroad just takes a bit more planning with diabetes. I make sure that I have enough supplies for an extra week or two in case flights are delayed, or I drop an insulin cartridge, take syringes with me in case my pen breaks and extra blood strips in case I get sick and need to do more tests. I carry everything in my hand luggage, as I know I won't be separated from it. Airport security always makes me feel a bit nervous, but I've only been asked to open my bag once, and when they saw my injection pen they just waved me through. Once I was on a flight where the meal had not been put on the plane. I told the crew I had diabetes and they each gave me something from their lunches. It was a bit embarrassing. I now always make sure I take some food with me on the plane.

(Nicola, 30)

I love travelling and have been to South Africa for three months, inter-railing throughout Europe twice as well as on holiday to Africa on several occasions, Central America and Thailand. I often give friends or my husband a small supply in case mine is lost or stolen. Time zones are quite difficult. I just try and inject on UK time for my longer-acting insulin and amend the shorter-acting for whenever meal times are. Heat is difficult as it mucks around with your insulin and I definitely should have invested in some sort of cool bag as it seems to work at half the power if it gets too hot. It's not a big deal, you have to see it as part of the organisation before and during the trip. However it's annoying that even if you plan ahead it can disarm you quite easily.

(Jane, 34)

I went travelling for 13 months on my own. I never thought it would be possible to go but it was so much easier than I thought it'd be. If you think about it too much you'd never go. I got cool bags to keep my insulin in and took loads of spares and split my insulin between two bags. I always had one pen on me. My best moment was snorkelling on the Great Barrier Reef.

(Jason, 27)

Once when I was on holiday in Turkey my insulin had gone cloudy and not right due to the heat. My Mum remembered a rather mad idea from the diabetic nurse; fill a sink with cold water, soak a pair of knickers in the cold water and wrap the insulin inside, leave in sink and throughout the day top up with more cold water. I lived to tell the tale!

(James, 28)

Q I am worried about Ali going to university; how will she manage her diabetes with the pressures of being away from home?

A Leaving home is probably the first time young people will take over full responsibility for everything, including their diabetes. There are bound to be mistakes, but this is part of their learning process. It's their time to decide how they want to live and manage in their adult life. All you can do is to let them know you are there for them.

There will be things that come up, like where to store insulin, remembering to renew prescriptions as well as managing with late nights and alcohol. If you worry too much this may make your child more anxious than is necessary.

Remember that when they go away from home there will be so many exciting new adventures. If every time you speak to them you ask about their diabetes, rather than their accommodation, their course or their new friends they may get annoyed with you and feel you don't trust them and are not interested in anything else other than their diabetes.

At university I was worried about where to keep my insulin. There was a common fridge and I knew if I left it there I'd have to tell everyone but if they didn't know what it was it'd be thrown out. So I got a little fridge for my room.

(Jason, 27)

Looking after myself 24/7 was fine. In fact, it was quite refreshing to get on with it myself. My mum would often ring me up and the first thing she would ask me was, 'How are your sugars?', and I'd often get really irritated by it. I know she only cares but it did really get on my nerves. I don't want to be asked all the time what my blood sugars are. I'm Juliet, not Juliet the diabetic.

(Juliet, 22)

When I went to college, at first I didn't tell anyone and I'd go to the toilet to inject, I just got on with it.

(Mike, 27)

Q **Will diabetes have an impact on choosing or holding down a chosen job?**

A With diabetes, the only thing stopping someone is chaotic blood glucose levels. As explained at the start of this chapter, most jobs are not limited by diabetes, even those involving emergency care where good awareness to hypos and stable blood glucose levels are needed. With all the different insulin regimens available there should be something to suit everyone if there is enough motivation to try.

If you are worrying about this issue be careful your child doesn't pick up on it and limit their options. It might make you feel better if your child chooses one particular job but it is your child's life and they need to feel fulfilled and live with their choices long after you are around.

Once at work, it seems sensible to tell one person at work about your diabetes, but this has to be a personal decision; there is no legal obligation to tell employers or fellow employees. As discussed in previous chapters, how people without diabetes have reacted in the past to your child having diabetes can determine how and when they want to tell work colleagues. They may not want everyone to know they have diabetes as the first and only thing about them. This is usually more of a worry than a reality unless they make a big deal about their diabetes themselves.

I tell who I need to at work but not on the first day, only after they've got to know me, so if they see me eating they know it's not because I'm greedy.

(Mike, 27)

I don't tell work colleagues about my diabetes. It's not a big deal to me but it looks like it is to others. When they find out about it they worry and everything you do is, 'Is everything OK?' I don't want people constantly worrying and I don't want it to be a reason for anything. But if I do have a hypo and they don't know I'm diabetic they might think my behaviour's a bit erratic.

(Jason, 27)

I always tell people at work about my diabetes. Lack of understanding is always there, but you get used to it. I've never had any negative reactions, usually its quite funny how wrong people are. For example, often people ask, 'Are you the diabetic that can eat cake?' I'm a trainee teacher and at school I usually tell my class. Children understand better than adults, its surprising.

(James, 28)

Diabetes has never got in the way of work for me. All reactions I've had to my diabetes at work have been very positive and I feel like I can talk about it very openly and do my injections at my desk no worries. I usually find that I'll just check my blood sugars in front of them and most of the time people are like 'Oh, you have diabetes' or 'What's that?' Then I explain. I don't really like bringing it up just out of the blue unless I have to.

(Juliet, 22)

I tell people at work but quite casually and they are always intrigued but the subject doesn't come up much.

(Jane, 34)

Q Should my child expect problems from potential partners in accepting their diabetes?

A Many young people as well as parents worry about future boyfriends and girlfriends. However, it is usually more of a worry than a reality. As a parent your worries for your child may cloud everything. Perhaps this may come from worry about who will look after your child when you are not here any more. Most parents just worry about their children, no matter what. There are always going to be a few 'bad eggs' out there, irrespective of diabetes. If you look at Chapter 11: The best and worst of times, you will read that many people with diabetes say their diabetes actually sparks conversation and can be a good talking point. Others use it as a test of the person they are going out with. It doesn't make sense if a person doesn't accept another because of their diabetes, but it can be a concern for a young person with diabetes, particularly for those who have had limited experience of relationships. Many people worry about relationships anyway until they meet their soulmate and then nothing else really matters anyway.

Everyone has their own individual style as to when and how to tell their partner they have diabetes and this will likely change with age, moulded by previous experiences. It is only natural for the partner without diabetes to worry a bit if they don't know anything about diabetes, especially if little information is shared with them. They may then search on the internet and find frightening statistics which are irrelevant to the individual.

I told my husband pretty much straight away but then I was pretty sure about my feelings for him so it was worth being open. The older you get the less embarrassed you feel.

(Jane, 34)

When it comes to relationships, when do you tell someone? You don't want it to be a big deal but if you avoid it, it looks like one. Diabetes is only a big thing if you make it a big thing.

When I was younger I felt awkward, especially if I'd known a person as a friend first and hadn't told them. It can look as if you're hiding something. When I meet someone and we're chatting about so many things I wouldn't want diabetes to be the focus. Now I just drop it into conversation, but when I was younger I did make a big thing about it. One girlfriend used to get cross 'cos I had a lot of night hypos. I was a bit pissed off about it, it wasn't my fault.

When I had my first serious relationship, it did freak me out about getting complications and popping off early. I thought, what if something went wrong with my diabetes and I don't hang around for them? But I stopped worrying, there's a million and one things that could happen in your life.

(Jason, 27)

I've had three long-term relationships. I don't usually mention my diabetes if I'm dating someone casually. My diabetes has never been a big deal. I'd never hide it, or do an injection under the table.
Various boyfriends have seen me completely out of it. Then they'll be constantly anxious for a couple of weeks after. My partner worries about me on a day-to-day basis. we've talked about complications, but he says he doesn't care. He'll love me no matter what.

(Katherine, 30)

I have always told boyfriends about having diabetes straight away because it's something important about me. I've always thought that if someone reacted badly to finding out I had diabetes then they weren't worth knowing. Mostly people have taken their cues from me. Because I'm open about it, but make it clear that I'm the one that manages it, I tend to get the sort of response I need: looking out for me, not nagging and wanting to know more about it.

(Nicola, 30)

Usually, it is a nice positive and curious reaction I get from partners. If they take time to find out about my diabetes and try to help me as much as they can then I like that. If they care about my diabetes, then they obviously care about me, so it's a good sign.

Having sex has never really been an issue with my diabetes. I've only had sex with a boyfriend that knows me well and I joke about having my sugar tablets next to my bed just in case I go hypo. I did have an insulin pump for six months which did get in the way of sex a little bit. However, I had a very nice and supportive boyfriend at the time and before we 'did it' I just unattached myself. It was quite funny hearing the pump bleep every few minutes because it was disconnected.

I think it's very important to have a boyfriend that is supportive of your diabetes. I find that if I am with someone that genuinely cares about me, they will take an interest and care for me and my diabetes. I have been with someone who never really gave a crap about my diabetes, if I had a high blood sugar and was upset they didn't really show much interest. It then made me wonder whether they had much interest in me at all.

(Juliet, 22)

I've not had any problems with partners finding out about me being diabetic. My only worry is that when I am low and I have to eat my boyfriend thinks I am being greedy.

(Bridget, 32)

Q **Is it difficult having children if you have diabetes?**

A It shouldn't be any harder to have children, but the associated problems with having diabetes with high blood glucose levels can cause problems to both the mother and the child. Like everything to do with diabetes, planning and organisation are important. You will need to take 5 mg folic acid daily before conceiving and for the first 12 weeks of pregnancy. Many healthcare professionals become frustrated with patients who will suddenly, remarkably, manage extremely tight blood glucose levels when trying to have a baby and during pregnancy, when it seems to have been impossible to achieve before. However, for those with diabetes, a wanted pregnancy is a motivation and a short-term goal that can be achieved.

There is a lot of guilt wrapped up in having diabetes. There is the guilt that you as parents feel but also guilt from those with diabetes when eating sweet foods or having high blood glucose levels. There is also guilt in the thought of harming an unborn child because of high blood glucose levels. For some, the motivation and effort needed for tight blood glucose control for the rest of their life feels too much, and they prefer to use their energies on other things, like socialising or their career. During pregnancy, women with diabetes have a lot of input from health professionals and this also provides some of the much-needed support for the motivation that is demanded. This level of input is not available for everyone in other circumstances, so it is not surprising that at other times blood glucose levels are not as tightly managed.

I'd feel guilty if my children had diabetes.

(Flin, 23)

Becoming pregnant, giving birth to a new child and bringing up children is both exciting and rewarding, as well as extremely hard work - even more so with diabetes in your life. As long as you have good blood sugar control, there shouldn't be any complications. With this in mind, it is advisable to plan your pregnancy at least 6 months before you conceive, to ensure your blood sugar levels are well controlled. Once pregnant, keeping tight control of your blood sugars is not easy, although it is achievable. I tested my blood sugar often, on a regular basis, and recorded the results so I could see any patterns to try to predict the amount of insulin required and when it is needed before losing control.

During each trimester, insulin requirements increase. A plus point of being a 'diabetic mum-to-be' is that you will have several scans throughout the nine months. This can be both exciting and fascinating as you watch your baby grow and develop into a recognisable 'little person'. This can help with the 'bonding' of you and your baby even before it's been born. The scans are also a very good motivational tool to ensure blood sugars are kept controlled.

As a woman living with diabetes for 23 years and having had four children, this has given me a strong sense of responsibility to keep my blood sugars tightly controlled as I have others depending on me. It can be the most frightening experience to go into a hypo when you have your children with you. It's not only upsetting for me but also for my young children to witness.

(Beth, 34, wife and mother to four children)

As soon as you are aware you're having a baby it's all about diabetes. I was so focused that I wanted to have a healthy baby I was testing 20 times a day. I was always planning - I always knew what I was doing.

(Lucia, 37, wife and mother)

I used to feel really anxious about whether I'd be able to have children or not. When I was newly diagnosed someone told me that diabetes would prevent me from being able to. Recently I spoke to my diabetes doctor and nurse about it. They explained that the main challenge is keeping really good blood sugar control during pregnancy and 6 months beforehand. There is always an element of doubt or anxiety in my mind, but since speaking to my clinic I am feeling really positive and hopeful about having kids in the next few years.

(Nicola, 30)

I would love to be a parent and my diabetes would not stop this.

(James, 28)

I would love to be a parent and have no more worries than my female friends who wish to become mothers. I think if there are any problems I will deal with it when it happens.

(Bridget, 32)

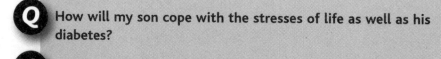

Q How will my son cope with the stresses of life as well as his diabetes?

A Life can be stressful at times anyway, with or without diabetes. However, there is an extra burden with having diabetes whichever way you look at it – whether it is just the extra time factor involved,

A continued

high or low blood glucose levels, injections, food restraints, worry or dealing with other people's attitudes. Learning how to juggle the demands of life is a necessary part of becoming an adult. Those of us who have diabetes have to learn how to look after ourselves and do everything everyone else has to do as well. It is perfectly manageable with a good routine. There may be times when it seems to be more than a nuisance, as discussed in Case 1, especially if routine is not part of that person's desired life. It has been a common theme throughout the book that diabetes can be used as a weapon if someone feels angry or out of control. With better blood glucose control, those with diabetes feel healthier, both in mind and body. Because they can cope better they can actually do more.

Support from friends and family is important for all of us. Being able to talk and share feelings is key to easing a burden through feeling understood. It doesn't make problems go away, but it can help individuals feel that they are being understood. This can be easier said than done if you are not the sort of person who is used to opening up, but once you are aware of it, you can practise. If you start the process of talking and sharing how you feel about things you will see that those who you share it with often follow suit. Whilst this may seem hard when you are communicating with your children, it is worth the investment of trying. If trying on your own seems too hard there are many support agencies that can help you with these skills. I use the word 'skill' because communication is something that can be improved with practice, like a muscle that needs to be warmed up before it is ready to be used.

I still struggle now; I find it difficult to write down my bloods. My HbA$_{1c}$ is good so on the surface everything's fine. It's difficult to pinpoint down what needs improving in an appointment every six months. Stress does affect my blood sugars a lot but sometimes I don't realise it. With me it brings me lower.

(Flin, 23)

Sometimes I do get down about having to be extra careful. Sometimes when I'm out it seems that everyone has no worries, no cares and I have to go to the loo and do my insulin again. And sometimes my sugars are low and I have to take some time out and eat my dextrose tablets or my sugars are high and I have to deliberate whether or not to do a little injection, and if I don't I spend some of my night worrying and thinking, 'Ahhhh my sugars are really high right now' and I hate that.

(Juliet, 22)

What you can do

These points are also addressed to the young person involved, because by now you as a parent should have handed over much of the responsibility. However it may be useful to have a few of these suggestions at the back of your mind if your son or daughter likes to discuss things with you.

- **Talk to others who have been there, and done that.** Chances are, whatever seeming obstacle is causing concern, someone else has tried it before. This applies to anything from playing competitive sport to travelling across the world. Fellow like-minded people can be found through hospital clinics, young persons' support networks through charitable organisations or via the internet. Talking with someone who has been through the same thing may just serve as a springboard for ideas, but more importantly it will give your son or daughter the confidence to go for it. You will not do them any service by trying to discourage them from doing things and they may well end up resenting you for it instead.

- **Try not to focus solely on diabetes.** Ask your son or daughter about other aspects of their life before you ask about their diabetes, as their life is more than just diabetes. Although it may not feel like it, your life is more than looking after their diabetes too! If it doesn't feel like it, now may be your chance to regain some of your own life.

- **Trust your son or daughter to ask for help** or support when they need it, giving them the confidence they need to be independent.

Rachel's view

Even though I've always looked after my own diabetes, when I first left home there was a lot of new things to juggle – cooking for myself, washing, studying, boyfriends and managing my diabetes with alcohol, late nights and exam stress. It was always going to be a challenging time but it was also an exciting time for new adventure. Diabetes brought something new to balance.

I work in a hospital setting, looking after children who can become ill quickly. I need to make sure I am OK if I am to look after them and I am aware I need to be a good role model for those around me. Even so, many people at work are surprised I have diabetes. It never fails to amuse me and makes me wonder what their preconceptions are. I show them who I am. Rachel.

No two days are the same in my current job and I couldn't manage with good control if it wasn't for my insulin pump as it can allow for different activity levels and takes away the need to rely on eating at specific times. I do fewer blood tests at the weekends and when I'm not working to give myself a bit of a break.

Stress does affect my blood sugars. I really notice it when the stress is removed, such as on the first few days of a holiday when I completely relax – even if I'm doing nothing I have hypos all the time and then realise that I should have remembered from the last time to reduce my insulin.

When I first started working I didn't take into account that I needed to give myself extra time to manage my diabetes. I had always felt invincible. However, when there is limited time because of work it becomes noticeable that managing diabetes well does require time set aside to think about insulin doses and blood test results, as well as eating properly, staying fit, socialising and doing well at work. Having diabetes can also be tiring if blood sugars are up or down, not to mention the extra time it actually involves. I like my bloods to be just right so I can feel well and do more. Now I make that time because I have to and I have learnt the hard way when I thought I could do it all without stopping for breath. As a result I feel well whereas before I would be tired much of the time. Having said that, most of the time I just get on with it and people comment on my seemingly inexhaustible energy. I've also noticed that having diabetes is expensive – I dread to think how much I have spent on glucose tablets over the years and train tickets to hospital appointments. I haven't added it up as it might make me cross as I might have had a luxury holiday instead.

I used to be worried about having diabetes and having a family of my own. Meeting people like Beth, a mother of four, and Lucia, has inspired me to realise that it is possible. In fact, anything is possible, with or without diabetes.

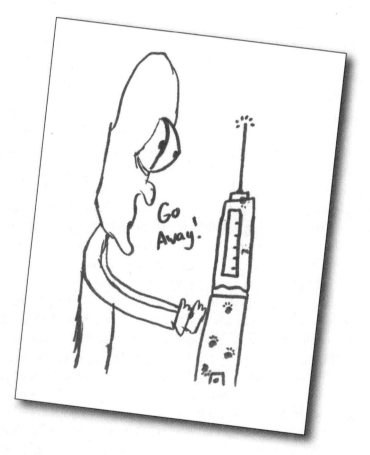

11

The best and the worst of times

This chapter comprises a series of questions and answers. I asked children and young people with diabetes, as well as adults who were diagnosed in childhood, a series of questions to help uncover their general feelings, hidden truths and cheeky moments about living with diabetes. I also asked some of the same questions to their parents. The answers speak for themselves and highlight the difference in priorities and worries that you have compared to your children.

What parents say

For many parents diabetes means a massive change that creeps into every corner of your life, especially at the beginning. Parents' worries often focus on the immediate: the hypos, injections and constant planning. You also worry about the future, feeling that you are unable to protect your child for ever. You worry about who will look after them when you cannot. Those of us with diabetes, however, mostly don't think about it a lot of the time, it just hits us occasionally. It is just one part of us and something that needs to be dealt with.

What the young people with diabetes say

For those with diabetes, it can be just one part of us, but it is also an inconvenience at times. When life is busy, diabetes can be an even bigger hassle, and it is easy to treat it as a punchbag as it is always close at hand. If diabetes is ignored over a long period and complications develop, then it can become more of a burden.

Each individual has a unique perspective that varies depending on current age and age of diagnosis, length of diabetes, parents' perspective, personality, presence or absence of complications and other outside factors. Attitudes often change with age and experience and can even fluctuate during a person's lifetime. The opinions given in this chapter are relevant to that individual only at the time when they are asked: a few years later, or at a different time, they may have answered differently. For example, young children often dislike injections and blood tests because of the physical aspect; older children find not eating sweets hard; teenagers may want to ignore the whole thing; and adults find it challenging to balance diabetes with the business of life. Children who are diagnosed when very young often do not remember life before diagnosis; it can be more 'normal' to them compared with those diagnosed later who have a clear memory of life before and after diagnosis. Adults who have complications appear to be either angry at not being given their best possible start as a child, or philosophical, rationalising that they preferred more liberal diabetes control even if this is connected with the onset of complications. Adults without complications often fear their onset and prefer to live a more disciplined life in order to avoid them.

The good and the bad

Most people can see a positive side to having diabetes. For young children this is centred on the things they feel they are not usually allowed, such as sweets when they are hypo. However, the reality is that they are not lucky to be in that situation in the first place. Adults with diabetes can see the benefits of regular health checks; they also seem to have an altered perspective which makes them more positive, appreciative and determined in life. In comparison, parents talk about health issues as being both positive and negative aspects of their child having diabetes. This sounds contradictory but highlights the parents' focus on the medical aspects of a child's diabetes. The issues surrounding growing up with diabetes are often in conflict. For example, how should you balance tight blood glucose control with being relaxed, but also worrying about complications? Should you give children treats but restrict them in other ways, such as with their food?

These differing attitudes between parent and child reflect all that is tied up in the anger, blame, guilt and frustration you feel when your child is diagnosed with diabetes. We get used to what needs to be done pretty quickly, and soon it becomes automatic. This is why for the person with diabetes, any worries or difficulties are often transient, coming and going; but for parents, your worries may be there a lot longer and may be more intense. Overall, life with diabetes needs only be a nuisance at its worst, but it seems clear that parents have some really bad times and worry a lot.

You may be rather surprised to hear all our diabetes-related excuses. These are inevitable; but should you let us get away with it? Well, some might say that there have to be some perks. I used to be one of those people, but I believe this is a lazy answer. Yes, I have used the odd excuse myself, but in the long run it doesn't do any of us any favours. One of our biggest annoyances is other people's reactions to and misunderstandings of our diabetes. If we are using diabetes to con our way out of situations we are only reinforcing these prejudices. Initially I did consider omitting the confessions from this chapter but felt that if I did I would also be complicit. So, I feel I must apologise to my fellow 'diabetic' friends when I recommend you do not let your child use their diabetes as an excuse. This is particularly relevant to children at school because it is easy for children to recognise who is not 'in the know' and fool them. It is especially satisfying to be able to 'get one over' on teachers.

Finally, please take note of the advice about having diabetes, straight from the expert mouths of your children, whose experience spans more than 30 years.

Q **What does having diabetes mean to you?**

A Answers from children, young people and adults with diabetes

I try to make it as small a part of my life as possible.
(Luke, 17)

I'm no different to everyone else. I just have to take medicine before meals.
(Margaret, 12)

I've got to do injections and blood tests. It's part of me. It doesn't faze me in the slightest.
(Nigel, 37)

It doesn't seem like anything to talk about.
(Janina, 13)

continued on next page

A continued

I do resent it totally. It's frustrating and a pain in the arse to cope with.
(Beatrice, 31)

Everything really. Whenever you eat something you have to look at the carbs. You have to take injections. If you're not diabetic you have more fun. I have to look after myself in case something might happen to me and take caution with my health.
(Kiet, 16)

Diabetes is simply part of everyday life and part of me. I can't imagine life without diabetes.
(Nicola, 30)

The added health issue but other than that I forget about it and get on with my life.
(George, 35)

Sometimes I have to be responsible for myself. If my Mum's not around it's just me — I have to know what to do.
(Jeffrey, 9)

Hospitals.
(Martina, 28)

I can't ever imagine life without diabetes. It's difficult to know how I'd be without it. Many people think I'm quirky and funny to be around. Much of that is because of my diabetes. I'm able to laugh at life. I enjoy life as much as possible – that's a reflection of my perspective. I don't resent my diabetes, it's just something I've got. It's not going to change, so you have to deal with it, otherwise you've wasted your life. It's not the easiest thing to cope with growing up.
(Jason, 27)

A *continued*

Being different but not wanting to feel different. It makes you a lot different to everyone else. I wanted to be normal. I spent years making sure everything I did was normal.

(Susie, 24)

A controlled life, a healthy life. I don't feel I am any different.

(Rebecca, 35)

It helps you in a way because it helps you to control your diet. It's like a maze that has no end, but then you soon learn how to cope with the stress.

(Alex, 12)

Not as much as it used to. It used to be a big thing and something I worried about a lot.

(Katherine, 30)

A lot different now than it used to, I've grown into it.

(Ruth, 38)

It doesn't mean anything to me. I can't differentiate between having it and not.

(Flin, 23)

It's depressing at times when all your friends are eating sweets and you can't have anything but it can be a bit rewarding at other times.

(Maeve, 9)

Diabetes to me is quite private. My friends and family know I am diabetic but day to day I generally forget my diabetes and continue with my life.

(Bridget, 32)

Q What does having diabetes mean to you?

A Answers from parents

- Constant worry
- Amy [4 years] will be different, nothing will be impossible but things will be harder. It feels like I will never get a day off again. I've got to be organised about eating, no more snacking throughout the day without a 'proper' meal. I'm coming to realise you don't 'control' diabetes you 'manage' it as best you can and try not to get too hung up on readings.
- On a good day it's just another thing. On a bad day it's utterly horrible.
- A 'life change' for her, me and all those who interact with her. I feel that the spontaneity of life has somewhat gone and perhaps we do not have the carefree attitude that we once had. Everything has to be organised and disciplined within all areas.
- A whole new lifestyle for the rest of my daughter's life. She must think constantly about her condition in whatever it is she is doing. It also means having to watch carefully and to maintain and control her diet, constantly monitor her blood sugar level to ensure her diabetes management is absolutely the best it can be to negate any future complications.
- I have to allow this medical condition into all our lives but not let it take over.
- He is my son first. As it's been eight years this October it's now the norm. It's other people who need educating, as they are scared and confused about how to treat him.
- Having to be organised. Making sure I have all the supplies necessary like injections, needles, Hypostop gel, drinks, snacks, etc. Continuous – every day of every week of every year. Being regulated by the clock for breakfast/lunch/tea. Never having a day off or a holiday.
- Most of the time diabetes means a pain in the arse! All the extra planning and worrying and then things still go wrong!!! I don't let it stop Sam [4 years] from doing things that other kids his age do,

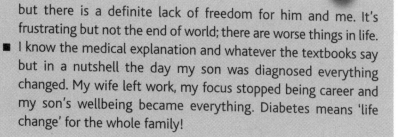

A *continued*

but there is a definite lack of freedom for him and me. It's frustrating but not the end of world; there are worse things in life.

■ I know the medical explanation and whatever the textbooks say but in a nutshell the day my son was diagnosed everything changed. My wife left work, my focus stopped being career and my son's wellbeing became everything. Diabetes means 'life change' for the whole family!

Q What's the best thing about having diabetes?

A Answers from children, young people and adults with diabetes

I get to go to lunch early.

(Darren, 12)

There's no good thing about having diabetes. There are some positives, such as my motivation and focus with competitive sports, but I will never say it's good to have diabetes, of course it's not.

(Nigel, 37)

Having chocolate before PE.

(David, 11)

Sweets when you're low.

(Leo, 10)

Being more self-aware about your body and how to look after yourself. More healthy than I'd otherwise be. I get regular check-ups.

(Beatrice, 31)

Becoming more independent earlier. It's made me become more organised.

(Susie, 24)

continued on next page

A continued

I'm healthy and have a great social life as I have made some brilliant friends through my voluntary work related to diabetes. A long life compared to others.

(Rebecca, 35)

The Disability Living Allowance.

(Luke, 17)

You get to go on special diabetic holidays and meet new friends who have the same condition as you.

(Margaret, 12)

I get away with a lot of stuff at school.

(Janina, 13)

It can become a good conversation piece.

(George, 35)

I can't think of anything. It's not exactly what you'd call good.

(Jeffrey, 9)

It makes you learn to be completely in touch with your body, emotionally and physically.

(Martina, 28)

If there was something wrong it would come up in my routine checks.

(Mike, 27)

A continued

It helps you to be more aware of what's going on in your body and what you eat.

(Alex, 12)

It's given me a different perspective to other people, some who are oblivious living their stress-free life.

(Jason, 27)

It's made me a stronger and more organised character and someone who doesn't waste chances.

(Katherine, 30)

Nothing really.

(Kiet, 16)

It gives you an excuse to be healthy. When they're handing round cakes at work I can say, 'No thanks, I can't', even though I could.

(Ruth, 38)

At school I used to get out of things. If I needed a breather I'd just put up my hand and the teachers just said, 'Yes, whatever', assuming it was because of my diabetes. It was nice to be different.

(Flin, 23)

The best thing is being able to have coke or lemonade in class when I have a hypo and sweets before PE.

(Maeve, 9)

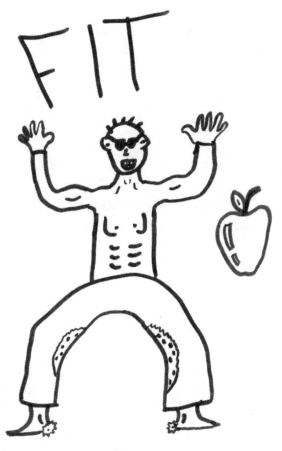

Fit!

Q **What's the best thing about having diabetes?**

A Answers from parents

- She takes care of her health.
- There is no best thing about diabetes but I have to admit the 'no queuing' armband at Alton Towers at Easter was such fun and getting into the local cinema free of charge is great too! [www.ceacard.co.uk is the website for the Cinema Exhibitors Association Card – which you can get if you are in receipt of Disability Living Allowance. It

A continued

entitles the holder of the card to one free ticket for a person accompanying them to the cinema.]

- We do spend a lot of time together, she will probably eat the best diet out of everyone in our house, and it makes me eat better as I now sit down with her more often so my diet has improved. Does it make her 'special'? I'm not sure, as she was always special but more cherished perhaps.

- This is a hard question to answer. I'm not sure I would describe it as 'best' but the positives are that we appreciate each other and our health much more now – we were close anyway but we make even more time for our children now. It has also led to us meeting some truly inspiring people.

- Personally, selfishly, I gave up work – I hated it at first but have come to love my new role as housewife, mother, school volunteer, dog walker and domestic goddess. It's great. My son will be stronger and braver and more secure. We are definitely a stronger family because of this.

- The message of healthy eating, looking after your health, promoting exercise is all good stuff. I also feel that when a person is faced with a condition or issue it does make them a stronger person, it makes that person question more and they are able to face the condition with a determined attitude.

- Loads. I had to stop being selfish and think of the family not myself. I now try to make decisions based on their needs not mine! I also think my sons and I are closer as we have all been through so much.

- I am more aware of what my son eats and I keep the sugar intake lower than I probably would. I think (hope) it will probably make him a stronger person longer term.

- He gets to go on holidays and see places that he might not see like a once in a lifetime trip to EuroDisney with the hospital.

- I find it difficult to see anything being good about my daughter having a life-long medical condition from an early age. It still seems very unfair. The complications and long-term effects scare me.

- The best thing is that he will (hopefully) grow up a lot healthier and more aware of how to care for his body than most people his age.

Q **What's the worst thing about having diabetes?**

A Answers from children, young people and adults with diabetes

Being called 'biscuit boy' at school.

(David, 11)

When people ask you loads of questions.

(Margaret, 12)

Being at the back of the dinner queue and not having as many Easter eggs.

(Leo, 10)

Being different as a child. It doesn't bother me so much now.

(Nigel, 37)

Injections.

(Darren, 12)

Dealing with other people's ignorance and having to eat when you're not hungry

(Lizzie, 27)

It's an inconvenience. You always have a hypo at the wrong time ...the only time you need a good sleep you wake up at 2 in the morning...or if you're in a rush, you have a hypo.

(Mike, 27)

Not being able to join the army.

(George, 35)

When I go high - it makes me lethargic, tired and lazy. It's not good for my school work.

(Luke, 17)

A continued

Not being able to eat a lot of sweets. My friends are always eating sweets. I have to watch them eating them, it gets irritating.

(Chantelle, 12)

Not being able to have a day off.

(Susie, 24)

Having to do an injection before you eat.

(Margaret, 12)

Fear of complications.

(Beatrice, 31)

When you go to the streets to buy food and see your friends eating — it makes you angry. You have to take injections before eating.

(Kiet, 16)

People asking strange unnecessary questions and getting the facts wrong, like, 'If you collapse shall I do your injection?'

(George, 35)

If my sugar goes low I might go into a hypo.

(Jeffrey, 9)

It debilitates you sometimes and can be debilitating.

(Martina, 28)

Diabetes is always with you, day in, day out. It means that if you are having a bad time for other reasons, diabetes feels like another thing to have to deal with.

(Nicola, 30)

continued on next page

A *continued*

Other people's completely uninformed perception. For example, that if I didn't inject I'd have a hypo, or when I'm asked, 'Have you still got it?' I think, 'Yeah, that organ hasn't started working yet'.

(Jason, 27)

The constant hypos and having to eat when I don't want to. Carrying extra supplies when going on holiday - finding space in the suitcase!

(Rebecca, 35)

Having to inject.

(Alex, 12)

Fear of complications in the future.

(Katherine, 30)

Having hypos and losing control. I look so stupid and I argue about stupid things. The edge of a hypo makes me scared as I don't know it's coming.

(Ruth, 38)

I get frustrated during sport, having to do a blood test and react to it, it's a pain. If I'm playing tennis and I have to stop, even if I use the finest needle it bleeds so much.

(Flin, 23)

The worst is having all the injections, you get used to it after a while but it can still really hurt.

(Maeve, 9)

Applying for a driving licence every three years; complications and laser treatment on my eyes; having hypos at really inconvenient times - during sex, in the middle of a gym session, giving a presentation at work.

(Bridget, 32)

Q What's the worst thing about having diabetes?

A Answers from parents

- She worries about her health.
- Never having a day off, you can't say we won't inject today, we'll lie in bed, eat chocolate for breakfast, dinner and tea. I think about it so many times a day whereas it only affects her at 'prickle' time. It is a bit of a weight on my shoulders and does get me down.
- Every time I drop him off somewhere I have to have a 'quick word' with the parent, carer or organiser. I have to stop myself from becoming controlling and neurotic.
- People's ignorance. The hypos are testing, even now seeing my daughter fighting and hitting me when low and refusing juice is stressful.
- The constant worry that everything is and will be OK; the future milestones and hurdles that will have to be overcome; teenage years, drinking, driving, pregnancy. I worry about my daughter and whether she is OK – I know that I can get a call at any moment.
- The inflexibility of having to carry test kits, snacks and drinks around all the time, and having to plan absolutely everything.
- Some sleepless nights and worry when he is ill.
- Hypos! Complications in later life; always having to be sensible. Injections up to six times a day, every day for the rest of her life. Fingerprick testing six times daily. Constantly having to explain that Type 1 is not because she's overweight or has eaten too many sweets. Not being able to just pop out. Always got to take a bag full of medical supplies. Making special arrangements. Being different from peers. Hypers.
- It's so unpredictable, no matter how much planning you do and when you think that you have thought of everything, somehow the sugar levels still end up too high or too low and either way my child ends up feeling crappy.
- Why him? Why our family? Why me? Is it my genes, have I given it to him? There is a lot of self-blame, as I could not stop it happening as a father.

Q Is there anything you worry about related to your diabetes?

A Answers from children, young people and adults with diabetes

Dying.

(Darren, 12)

I think about growing up and getting a job. They might not give me time to have a full lunch break.

(Margaret, 12)

The long-term effects and having a crash hypo in a busy place.

(George, 35)

If I grow up and I'm still diabetic it would be quite hard. Some people you go out with they might not know what was going on. You might not tell them 'cos you're hypo. They might take you to the hospital and they'll be like, I don't know 'cos he can't say anything.

(Jeffrey, 9)

Dying young. I don't want to die before I've done everything I want to do in life.

(Martina, 28)

Not really.

(Alex, 12)

I sometimes worry about the future and complications. I can feel guilty about times I haven't looked after myself as well as I could.

(Nicola, 30)

No.

(Jason, 27)

A continued

Leaving it too late to have children and the conceiving but I know the diabetes shouldn't give me problems.

(Rebecca, 35)

Having a hypo behind the wheel.

(Katherine, 30)

The complications. My blood sugar is higher than a normal person's. It's in my blood and going around me. The complications are just waiting to happen, waiting like a time bomb.

(Ruth, 38)

Nothing, you've just got to be careful.

(Flin, 23)

I would worry about really high blood levels and if my insulin doesn't go in right because if the insulin doesn't go right it produces a high reading.

(Maeve, 9)

Complications, which may arise as a result of my diabetes despite my best attempts at good diabetes control.

(Bridget, 32)

Q Is there anything you worry about related to diabetes?

A Answers from parents

- Her happiness and well-being.
- If I don't get 'good' control how she will be in later life when 'good' control is very difficult at the moment? Yes she will be able to have babies but again more difficult to start with without anything else going wrong.

continued on next page

continued

- Who will look after him when he is 80? Will somebody check his blood sugar for him?
- The threat of long-term complications – or finding him dead in his bed – absolutely terrifies me, so best not to think about it.
- When he has a severe hypo, ends up on a drip, isn't with it and is so ill my fear is he could go into a coma and die.
- Teenage years. Alcohol. Friends. Boyfriends. Complications. My daughter taking on the understanding and responsibility for her condition. She does not recognise when high or low which leads to some very scary incidents. How will she grow and develop?
- I fear that it has had an effect on our mother–son relationship, I'm not sure but I get the feeling that he may blame or resent me for it. My other worry is that he won't look after himself properly and suffer from lots of diabetes-related complications.
- My biggest fear is the hypo that requires a glucagon injection – I know I will be able to do it as it will be necessary but I hope I never have to. Another worry is that my daughter can't lead a 'normal' life in the usual sense – that everywhere she goes and in everything that she does, she needs to constantly think about her diabetes – her life is no longer as carefree as a teenager's should be.
- That he might not reach his full potential in an aspect of his life as he sees it.

Q Do you or have you ever used your diabetes to get your own way or as an excuse?

A Answers from children, young people and adults with diabetes

When I was younger I used to say 'my blood sugar is low' – it always happened when I was near a McDonald's.

(George, 35)

A continued

If I want a drink in class I say, 'I've got diabetes' and teachers say 'OK!' I put up my hand and say 'I have diabetes – I have to eat something'.

(Kaya, 12)

If I'm late for an appointment or work but actually I overslept and haven't got my arse out of bed!

(Beatrice, 31)

When my friends were smoking I used my diabetes as an excuse [not to start]. I used to say 'I don't know how it will affect my diabetes'.

(Mike, 27)

When you want to eat you just say you're low which can have benefits if you are hungry or in a rush.

(George, 35)

I used to hate Dextrose [glucose tablets to treat hypos]. I'd barter with the kids at school – I'd swap three Dextrose tablets for a chocolate bar. I don't know why they liked them, they tasted horrible. It's probably because they didn't have to eat them.

(Martina, 28)

In school when strict teachers would shout at me for eating in class I could just say 'I've got diabetes remember'. The look on their faces was always priceless!

(Nicola, 30)

When I went clubbing I could jump the toilet queue. I would waltz to the front of the queue with a friend saying 'I need to do my injection'. I felt a bit guilty but it was worth it!

(Susie, 24)

continued on next page

A *continued*

At school I used to say 'I don't feel very well, I'm having a hypo', to get out of PE classes.

(Rebecca, 35)

Sometimes if I'm late for work I say I had a hypo and couldn't get behind the wheel, when actually I slept in or have a hangover.

(Katherine, 30)

I once mentioned I was having a hypo in a boring clothes shop when I felt fine.

(Alex, 12)

It got me out of choir practice at school as I had to go home for a snack.

(Ruth, 38)

I blame my diabetes when I'm grumpy.

(Flin, 23)

When I have to go do a blood reading I get to miss five, ten minutes of class which in a way is good and bad, but still.

(Maeve, 9)

I sometimes say I have a diabetes clinic, when I don't, to leave work early.

(Bridget, 32)

Never, never, never. If you do that it embraces diabetes as a tool. However, other people try to use my diabetes for me. Sometimes people say, 'Can we get to the front of the queue because you're diabetic?' I say, 'we can jump to the front of the queue, but not because I'm diabetic'.

(Nigel, 37)

Q What would make life easier for you?

A Answers from children, young people and adults with diabetes

Taking a pill.

(Chantelle, 12)

Not being diabetic and winning the lottery.

(George, 35)

If I didn't worry.

(Jeffrey, 9)

If I could have a watch that constantly told me what my blood sugars are, and an instantly replenishing prescription cupboard would be useful too.

(Nicola, 30)

Knowing what blood sugar I was all the time.

(Jason, 27)

A wonderful bit of technology implanted inside the body that tests blood sugars for me!

(Rebecca, 35)

Not having diabetes, or at least not having to continuously monitor.

(Katherine, 30)

People listening. Instead of listening to the words and dismissing it, listening to what the actual problem was and thinking why there was a problem.

(Ruth, 38)

A watch to tell me what my blood sugar is.

(Flin, 23)

continued on next page

A *continued*

Nothing's hard with diabetes.

(Nigel, 37)

Well certainly taking away the injections but I know you always have to have them.

(Maeve, 9)

It would be good if everyone could experience a hypo then they would know what it feels like and may be a little more understanding.

(Bridget, 32)

Q **Do you have any particular bugbears?**

A Answers from children, young people and adults with diabetes

When people say 'You must be used to your injections by now'.

(Susie, 24)

The constant 'have you done this or that' like checking your blood or having done your injection. Mum still says 'There aren't a lot of carbs in that'. I hate it when people say 'You're lucky because you get to eat'. I think, 'I'd swap places with you'.

(George, 35)

People using diabetes as an excuse.

(Nigel, 37)

Having to inject in horrible environments, such as in dirty cafe toilets or having friends peering over your shoulder whilst injecting.

(Alex, 12)

A continued

I hate it when other people tell me how to manage my diabetes. It makes me feel like giving up or being 'naughty' just to prove them wrong. It also makes me angry when people complain about me doing my injection in front of them. I am always discreet about it, and I feel like saying 'sor-ry, at least you don't have to do it'. When I was younger I hated it when people called me 'a diabetic'. I can't stand labels and I always said 'I'm a GIRL, with diabetes'.

(Nicola, 30)

TV has not done a good job at dealing with diabetes issues and has only reinforced people's misunderstanding and prejudices. People don't understand it well enough. They tend to still have the 1980s view that you can't eat anything and diabetes is some horrific disease, which means you're abnormal.

(Jason, 27)

Other people eating my hypo food – the jelly babies are mine.' Also, when even the medical profession act surprised and say 'You don't look diabetic, you look so healthy'. I think, 'Do you expect it to be tattooed across my forehead? And I am healthy, I just have to inject four times a day.

(Katherine, 30)

I find it ridiculous that I can't see more than one health professional on the same day. It means I end up missing some appointments.

(Flin, 23)

continued on next page

When my husband and friends say, 'Have you done a blood test?' if they think I'm low. I just think, back off and let me deal with it myself. Also, when people don't offer me food because they assume I can't eat it. It's like, 'We know better than you what you want'.

(Ruth, 38)

Well yes, because sometimes we have parties at school and Brownies and everyone is having lots of crisps and sweets and Fanta, and I'm not allowed that sort of stuff and they wouldn't be able to do anything about it.

(Maeve, 9)

Q **Has your diabetes ever stopped you doing anything? Or have you ever been discriminated against because of your diabetes?**

A Answers from children, young people and adults with diabetes

Getting a pilot's licence, so now I skydive.

(George, 35)

Going to the Isle of Wight with school. Mum was like, 'Sorry Jeffrey, but no. It might be difficult going on a school trip. They might not really be OK. They might forget.'

(Jeffrey, 9)

Thankfully, no. It might even have made me more determined to do things I might not have otherwise done. Where I go, diabetes comes too, and I go where I like.

(Nicola, 30)

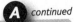
A continued

I used to do a regular aerobics class and had been going for years. There was a new teacher and she asked if anyone had a medical condition. I put my hand up and said I was diabetic and she told me in front of the whole class that I couldn't do the class. I replied that I'd been doing aerobics for five years and doctors recommend exercise. I had to leave class and never went back. It put me off telling other instructors about my diabetes. I'm in control of it and know my limits.

(Martina, 28)

Not now, but when I was at school I wasn't allowed to go on school trips due to lack of education and understanding with my parents and school. I used to tell friends I couldn't go because we couldn't afford it.

(Rebecca, 35)

I always wanted to join the army. On the entry form for the Territorial Army they asked 'Is there anything you suffer from?' I thought, 'No I don't', so I didn't write that I had diabetes. One training weekend I realised I had forgotten my insulin but I didn't want to tell the sergeant, as I would get kicked out. By the end of the weekend I ended up in hospital and was given a medical dismissal from the army.

(George, 35)

Camping with the Scouts at first, but once I became in control, I could manage. And now I camp quite frequently with no problem.

(Alex, 12)

Scuba diving.

(Jason, 27)

continued on next page

A continued

Once when I was a child my teacher couldn't get my sugar box open so she wouldn't let me go swimming. I had to sit on the side of the pool watching all my friends splash around. I still remember and I was 7.

(Martina, 28)

No.

(Katherine, 30)

Not because of my diabetes but because of my sight loss.

(Ruth, 38)

I wanted to do scuba diving in Australia and they wouldn't let me and I had to go snorkelling instead. I was really cross about it. They were being naive about diabetes and I did feel discriminated against. I was so cross with them that I went far away from the boat. I ended up seeing a shark, it was so close to me. I was travelling at the time and ended up going scuba diving in Malaysia instead.

(Flin, 23)

No, not in activity ways but in eating ways yes, because most foods have sugar or carbohydrates in them.

(Maeve, 9)

Getting driving and travel insurance.

(Bridget, 32)

Q What would you tell someone who had just been diagnosed with diabetes?

A Answers from children, young people and adults with diabetes

You're just the same as anyone else, there's nothing to worry about, you just have to inject before each meal. It's easy once you get used to it.

(Margaret, 12)

There are far worse things than having diabetes. Embrace it, live with it and conquer the world.

(Nigel, 37)

As you get more used to it, it gets easier and easier. Doing an injection every day is a bit like going to the toilet. It's not that bad once you get used to it.

(Kaya, 12)

It's important not to get hung up on one high reading. It's not the end of the world. Within reason don't let it stop you doing what you want to do. You just need to think extra hard.

(Beatrice, 31)

Look after yourself all the time. Don't get your diabetes involved in schoolwork. Enjoy life and don't keep thinking of diabetes. Don't be ashamed of having diabetes — you have a life to look forward to. Diabetes is just one thing you have to do.

(Kiet, 16)

Try your best to follow the basics and if you do eat sweets don't hide the wrapper, as they will be found! Be open with it.

(George, 35)

continued on next page

A continued

You shouldn't have a lot of sugary things or just a little bit.

(Jeffrey, 9)

Don't worry about it stopping you doing things. You can still have a fulfilling life as long as you learn how to work with it.

(Martina, 28)

Although it doesn't feel like it when you're first diagnosed, diabetes doesn't have to take over your life. If you respect it and work with it, and try not to resent it, it can be completely manageable. It's also natural to feel upset from time to time and you're not alone with that.

(Nicola, 30)

Understand what it means and how it works. Don't worry about it but don't forget about it either. Don't ever do anything different because you're diabetic. Do everything you want to do.

(Jason, 27)

Don't let it stop you living your life. It shouldn't stop you from doing what you want to achieve.

(Rebecca, 35)

It's a life-changing diagnosis but the advances that are happening means that it is not a life-shortening one.

(Katherine, 30)

Don't let it get to you, but also don't ignore it, you're in complete control of yourself.

(Alex, 12)

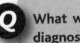

A continued

Listen to your doctor about the consequences in the future.

(Ruth, 38)

I wouldn't talk about diabetes unless they brought it up. I struggle to see it as 'it'.

(Flin, 23)

I would say just relax and get all the information you can get from your local doctor and find out about different sorts of insulin.

(Maeve, 9)

Be patient. Come to terms in your own time that you have diabetes but don't let it affect your life, otherwise you let diabetes take over your life rather than you living your life and letting the diabetes fit in around what you want to do.

(Bridget, 32)

Q What would you tell a parent of a child who has just been diagnosed?

A Answers from children, young people and adults with diabetes

It isn't as hard as it seems. It can be just like remembering to brush your teeth

(Alex, 12)

Don't go on at them and don't eat things that you think they shouldn't, as they will find a way around it.

(George, 35)

continued on next page

continued

It's hard to cope with but once you get a lot older and you'll be able to take care of yourself you'll get used to it.

(Jeffrey, 9)

Be supportive and help them without suffocating them in the way they lead their lives. Be understanding about what they are going through as a child, not what they are going through as a diabetic child. If they've got good control of their diabetes they're no different to anyone else.

(Nigel, 37)

I would explain how my parents helped me, as I feel they got it really right (for me at least). Little things helped like my sisters having Diet Coke so I wouldn't feel the odd one out. My parents were there for me, and even said they wished they could have diabetes instead of me. But the diabetes was always mine. What I ate, when I injected, how often I did blood tests, were all my decisions. Of course they were there in the wings, easing the burden, offering support, encouraging, enjoying the successes and sharing the downsides.

(Nicola, 30)

Don't focus on food all of the time. Give kids freedom with food. As soon as you restrict it, you want to do it more. Communicate with your child and try not to get angry and frustrated. Try to work with them.

(Martina, 28)

Your natural instincts are to micromanage your child's diabetes because you want to try to control it. You don't want anything bad to happen to your child and will do everything in your power to avoid those things. The reality is that your kid will have to grow up. The quicker they have to deal with it the better it is for them. Understand diabetes and know what you have to do but don't impose restrictions because of their diabetes.

(Jason, 27)

A continued

It's not the end of the world, a shock I know. Let your child lead a normal life as much as possible, don't stop them from going on school trips or activities as long as things are well planned and agreed with schools and club organisers. Let them understand the importance of looking after themselves but work together on this.

(Rebecca, 35)

Listen to your child. All children are going to rebel at some point and that means they are normal. You need to have a lower threshold for realising that when the blood glucose levels are going up it may actually be because of something the child has eaten – ask and the child may have the answer.

(Katherine, 30)

Listen to your child. Understand that as they grow up they might manipulate their diabetes to do things that they want to do. Get as much knowledge as you can about diabetes so when the doctors tell you something you follow it because you understand and not just because you are told to.

Make your child feel that they can tell you anything and that you'll understand. Don't say, 'No you can't' and instead try to understand why they're doing it. Back off a bit and try to empower your child to deal with it themselves. They have a bit of leeway to make mistakes. Don't frighten them about one-off high blood sugars.

(Ruth, 30)

continued on next page

A *continued*

Use the easiest spots for insulin first and then move on to the harder ones and don't really worry if your child has a blood reading like 16.7 because it isn't easy getting the right blood levels.

(Maeve, 9)

Do not blame yourself for your child developing diabetes, it is just one of those things. Give your child plenty of space to come to terms with having diabetes as they will be the ones who will have to do blood tests, inject, work out what food they are going to have, etc. Always be there to offer encouragement. If you have other children do not shut them out, encourage them to help their brother/sister if they have a hypo.

(Bridget, 32)

Q **What is the one thing you wish your parents had or hadn't done?**

A Answers from children, young people and adults with diabetes

I think they did a really good job.

(Jason, 27)

I wish they could have let up a bit on what I could and couldn't eat. It would have been better to have been listened to so that there could have been more understanding from my point of view.

(George, 35)

Have more confidence and knowledge to let me live my life more when I was younger. I would have liked to go on school trips.

(Rebecca, 35)

A continued

when I was diagnosed I had to stay in hospital an extra two days until my Dad had learnt how to inject an orange as he had a fear of injections.

(Katherine, 30)

Listening and giving me more credit for managing my diabetes myself.

(Ruth, 38)

I wish they wouldn't pester me to check my level.

(Alex, 12)

Panic. I remember my parents panicking when I was hypo and thinking, 'Why are they getting stressed out?' It made me think it was all because of me.

(Susie, 24)

Nothing, they were spot on. I was diagnosed in January and I was away next month on a school exchange programme to New York.

(Flin, 23)

Sometimes they nag me because of high blood levels like saying, have you been eating this or have you been eating that?

(Maeve, 9)

My parents couldn't have done any more or less – they were amazing and continue to be so!

(Bridget, 32)

Q How do you see your future with diabetes?

A Answers from children, young people and adults with diabetes

We'll still be together, me and my diabetes.

(Jason, 27)

I would want a cure for diabetics. I feel there is money to be made out of us and would like a cure soon.

(George, 35)

As I've just started pump treatment I am hoping to lead a normal life with regard to meal times - sleeping in at weekends, missing meals if I want to and better control during sport activities and not having to stuff my face with food.

(Rebecca, 35)

Positively; in the next 10 years there will be lots of exciting gadgets to monitor your blood sugar. I'm just buying extra time until it becomes a reality.

(Katherine, 30)

I live from day to day and live my life to the full as much as possible. I know that life is special, precious and what's important.

(Ruth, 38)

I see me in my house cooking, weighing all my food and giving myself insulin looking all stressed and that's if I have kids!

(Maeve, 9)

A continued

I'll be injecting for the rest of my life. My Mum reads about all the latest research. It never quite works out. It always seems to come and go. I'm accepting. I don't feel the need to talk about things; I just want to get on with it.

(Flin, 23)

Controlled.

(Alex, 12)

Continuing the same as now. I don't worry about the future – what will be will be.

(Bridget, 32)

My future will be what I make of it, irrespective of my diabetes. I am living my future now - happy, fulfilled and doing what I want and need to do.

(Rachel, 32)

Who's who

Many children, young people and adults have contributed to this book. Any names that appear have been changed to allow individuals to speak openly and to protect their privacy. More contributed than could be included in these pages, but all are remembered and valued; where contributions do not appear it is because a similar feeling has been voiced elsewhere in the book.

In the preceeding chapters, contributors have talked about nothing but diabetes. Here is a taste of who they are.

Aiden, 9, diagnosed aged 4

Aiden loves all sports, playing the cornet and spending time with his brother and friends. He also loves writing stories – he has a great imagination – and telling jokes to his classmates. When he grows up he wants to be an author or a comedian.

Alex, 12, diagnosed aged 11

Alex likes archery and wants to join the police force when he is older. He says, 'I won't let my diabetes stop me from doing anything'.

Amanda, 9, diagnosed aged 6

Amanda loves her gymnastics, dancing and learning French. She is enjoying learning to play the piano and is preparing for her Grade 1 exam next term.

Anna, 13, diagnosed aged 12

Anna is sports-mad: she has represented her county in hockey and also attends clubs for trampoline, tennis and dancing. You'd think that would take up all her spare time, but she also enjoys hanging out with friends and loves to shop.

Beatrice, 31, diagnosed aged 14

Beatrice works as a training manager, which involves lots of presentations and travelling the globe. She enjoys safari trips to far-flung places, which often involve camping in the bush at night and trekking up mountains. She keeps herself fit with regular aerobic classes and visits to the gym.

Beth, 34, diagnosed aged 12

Beth is a sociable character who enjoys nothing better than a glass of wine and a chinwag with her close friends. She enjoys a busy family life with her husband and four children, gardening and charitable activities. She lives life to the full.

Bridget, 32, diagnosed aged 17

Bridget enjoys swimming, keeping fit, listening to music, reading, wildlife and conservation, going to the cinema and theatre, walking and attending concerts. She ran her first London Marathon last year and is planning on walking the Coast-to-Coast path in June to raise funds for St Luke's Hospice in Sheffield. She currently works as a secretary at the University of Sheffield.

Chantelle, 12, diagnosed aged 10

Chantelle likes listening to music on her iPod and chatting to friends on social networking sites.

Charlotte and Debbie are both 27

and have been friends with Lizzie since primary school. Charlotte is a stylist and writer and Debbie is a handbag designer.

Daniel, 17, diagnosed aged 12

Watch out for Daniel – he's set to become a top graphic designer. He is at college at the moment studying graphic design and is on his way to university later this year. His main interests are in interior design, animation and any form of artwork. When he's not designing, you can normally find him either socialising on MSN or on the phone.

Darren, 12, was diagnosed earlier this year

Darren is a fast right-winger who likes to score goals. He is a massive Nottingham Forest fan and will always remain so, through thick and thin.

David, 11, diagnosed aged 9

David likes pool and table tennis, which he plays with his neighbour and older brother Richard.

Flin, 23, diagnosed aged 9

Flin is in training to run the London Marathon next year. He's mad on sport, having worked previously as a tennis coach. He still plays tennis regularly for a club and is also a keen footballer.

George, 35, diagnosed aged 9

George has spent time with the Territorial Army, and has worked for many years in jobs ranging from Security to being a Construction Foreman, as well as teaching key stage 1 and 2 Outdoor Activities. George loves adrenaline sports like climbing and skydiving and has 104 jumps under his belt. A big high was when he got to fly the plane at 13,000 ft.

Guy, 33

Guy, 33, is Lizzie's brother He works in adult education and enjoys swimming, horse riding, cooking and watching any type of sport. He was recently married.

Jane, 34, diagnosed aged 9

Jane is an Exhibitions Officer in an art gallery, enjoys hiking, travel and reading.

Janina, 13, diagnosed aged 7

Janina has recently passed her Grade 2 clarinet with Distinction, enjoys gymnastics, writing stories and is in all the top sets at school.

James, 28, diagnosed aged 3

James works as a Newly Qualified Teacher and support worker for young adults with learning difficulties. He loves Doctor Who, his many cats and enjoys trips away with friends, having recently visited Switzerland and Greece.

Jason, 27, diagnosed aged 7

Jason is a Senior Consultant to a major retailer in the UK and was recently awarded a National Award for Best Use of Data in Retail. He has spent 13 months travelling around the world on his own and knows how to have a good time.

Jeffrey, 9, diagnosed aged 4

Jeffrey is mad about football. He is a right mid-fielder in the school team and probably wants to play football professionally when he is a bit older. He trains twice a week and has weekly matches. He is also particularly good at maths.

Juliet, 22, diagnosed aged 17

Juliet enjoys spending time with friends, playing netball, and taking long walks by the beach. Her new job working for a Japanese company in London means trying out lots of authentic Japanese restaurants.

Katherine, 30, diagnosed aged 9

Katherine is rather a busy bee. Not only is she a General Practitioner in London, she is also busy starting up a community art gallery whilst writing a novel.

Kaya, 12, diagnosed aged 10

Kaya has recently learnt how to throw a pot on a potter's wheel in school. She has just finished her first bowl which she made for her Mum's birthday and painted it in stripes of different colours.

Kiet, 16, diagnosed at 15

'Music is my life', says Kiet, who plays the keyboard and wants to be a Music Producer in the future. He also enjoys hanging around with friends and generally having fun in life.

Leo, 10, diagnosed aged 5

Leo enjoys endless games of chess with his brother and represented his school at the county championships aged 7 when he won first place. He used his prize money to buy a paint set.

Liam, 12, diagnosed aged 3

Liam has always enjoyed making things, whether it's paintings or helping his Mum in the kitchen cook the Sunday roast.

Lizzie, 27, diagnosed aged 8

Lizzie used to play goalkeeper at school and still likes to be at the centre of fun. She enjoys crossing continents on different modes of transport, be it bicycle, donkey, boat or something more conventional.

Lucia, 37, diagnosed aged 5

Lucia works as a Customer Service Manager for an Awarding Body in the City. She recently married and lives with her husband and their lively 7-year-old boy who is her pride and joy. Lucia is about to embark on a career change and commence full time education in September to become a Montessori teacher.

Luke, 17, diagnosed aged 15

Luke is working towards his A-levels and plans on studying Psychology at university. He is a keen musician, playing the drums and violin.

Maeve, 9, diagnosed aged 7

Maeve loves lots of different things – she plays the saxophone, enjoys singing, art and going to swimming lessons. Most of all, she likes reading and playing with her sisters on their Nintendo Wii.

Mai, 8, diagnosed aged 7

Mai is a keen rollerblader who has mastered jumping and can tackle those sharp corners! She also loves swimming, drawing and even writes poetry.

Margaret, 12, diagnosed aged 2

Margaret loves street jazz and performs every year at her local theatre, with costumes made by her Nan. Her favourite subjects at school are Art and Design Technology, in which she is currently making an electronic badge. Margaret is going to be a clothes designer when she is older.

Martina, 28, diagnosed aged 7

Martina lives a full life, doing all the things she wants, including singing, acting, travelling around, meeting new people, trying new sporting activities such as belly dancing and many other weird and wonderful things. Martina generally just loves life, people and new adventures.

Melanie, 27, diagnosed aged 15

Melanie works as a pharmaceutical rep, and has just returned from visiting gorillas in Rwanda. She enjoys playing badminton and tennis with family and friends.

Mike, 27, diagnosed aged 11

Mike is a primary school teacher and has just bought his first house. He studied music at college and is still a keen violinist.

Nicola, 30, diagnosed aged 11

Nicola works in Marketing, enjoys sailing holidays and is buying a house with her boyfriend this year.

Nigel, 37, diagnosed aged 3

Nigel used to be a professional athlete, having played rugby for his county and was offered a contract with Harlequins. Unfortunately a neck injury scuppered his plans to play rugby for England. Instead, he turned his hand to rowing and competed in the World Indoor Rowing Championships in 2000, when he was ranked seventh in the world for 10 000 metres. These days he is an agronomist (pest doctor), plays drums in a band and is a new dad.

Rachel, 32, diagnosed aged 9

Rachel is the book's author. She is a paediatrician with plans to improve diabetes care for children. Outside work, her big loves are dancing, especially salsa and modern jive. She has a passion for writing, both fiction and non-fiction, and when it's time to relax, you will find her playing her guitar with friends, walking by the sea or at the theatre.

Rebecca, 35, diagnosed aged 6

Rebecca is outgoing and lives life to the full. Time at work is spent as a Quality Manager for a Telecommunications Company. In her spare time she loves being with her family, having weekends away, and also enjoys sport, gardening and dancing.

Ruth, 38, diagnosed aged 14

Ruth was recently married and works full-time in London.

Patrick, 4, diagnosed aged 2

Patrick is a big Dr Who fan. He likes show and tell at school and recently brought in a Dr Who magazine and a Ben 10 Omnitrix watch. He also loves gymnastics and football.

Summer, 13, diagnosed aged 2

Summer has a great sense of fashion and loves trampolining.

Susie, 24, diagnosed aged 8

Susie works for a community arts organisation and is always on the go. She loves anything creative even though much of her time at work is spent in meetings! She has loads of friends who she likes cooking experimental dishes for and taking to the theatre.

Tom, 11, diagnosed aged 8

Tom loves listening to music and playing with his video games. He is mad on table tennis and plays for at least an hour a day (in the holidays) on his own tennis table in the basement of his house. He goes to the park a lot to play football and he plays for his school team.

Appendix:
Useful contacts

General

Diabetes UK
www.diabetes.org.uk
Tel: 020 7424 1000

Disability Rights Commission
www.drc-gb.org
Tel: 0845 604 6610 (England)
Tel: 0845 604 8810 (Wales)
Tel: 0845 604 5510 (Scotland)
For advice on allowances,
employment and discrimination.

International Society for Paediatric
and Adolescent Diabetes (ISPAD)
www.ispad.org
Tel: +49 30 24603210

Juvenile Diabetes Research
Foundation (JDRF)
www.jdrf.org.uk
Tel: 020 7713 2030

Websites for children, teenagers and young adults with diabetes

www.t1kids.org.uk

www.diabetes.org.uk/Guide-to-diabetes/My-life

www.leedsth.nhs.uk/sites/diabetes/teenage

Sexwise
www.ruthinking.co.uk
Tel: 0800 282930
Confidential advice on sex,
relationships and contraception
(general advice, not related to
diabetes).

Family Planning Association
www.fpa.org.uk
Tel: 0845 122 8690 (England)
Tel: 0845 122 8687 (Northern
Ireland)
Advice and help on contraceptive and
sexual health issues.

National Drugs Helpline
www.ndh.org.uk
Tel: 0800 77 66 00

Fast Forward
www.fastforward.org.uk
Tel: 0131 554 4300
Information on smoking, alcohol and
illegal drug use.

ChildLine
www.childline.org.uk
Tel: 0800 1111
For 24-hour advice on anything.

Parent support
www.childrenwithdiabetesuk.org
UK Children with Diabetes Advocacy

Group. Providing information and on-line support for families affected by diabetes in the UK. Mailing list forum provided by CWD Foundation Inc, USA.

www.childrenwithdiabetes.com (US equivalent)

Manufacturers

Abbott Diabetes Care UK
www.abbottdiabetescare.co.uk
Tel: 0500 467 466

ActavisUK Ltd
www.actavis.co.uk
Tel: 01271311 200

Advanced Therapeutics UK
www.advancedtherapeuticsuk.com
Tel: 01926 494 222

Animas
www.animascorp.co.uk
Tel: 0800 055 6606

Bayer Diabetes Care
www.bayerdiabetes.co.uk
Tel: 0845 600 6030

BBI Healthcare
www.bbihealthcare.com
Tel: 01792 229 333

BD Medical
www.bddiabetes.co.uk
Tel: 01865 781 510

Daiichi Sankyo UK
www.daiichi-sankyo.eu
Tel: 01753 893 999

Eli Lilly and Co
www.lilly.co.uk
Tel: 01256 315000

GlaxoSmithKline UK
www.gsk.com
Tel: 0800 221 441

Home Diagnostics
www.homediagnostics.com
Tel: 01489 569469

Merck Serono
www.merck-pharmaceuticals.co.uk
Tel: 020 8818 7200

Merck Sharp & Dohme
www.msd-uk.co.uk
Tel: 01992 467 272

Novartis Pharmaceuticals UK
www.novartis.co.uk
Tel: 01276 698 370

Novo Nordisk
www.novonordisk.co.uk
Tel: 0845 600 5055

Pfizer
www.pfizer.co.uk
Tel: 01304 616 161

Rosemont
www.rosemontpharma.com
Tel: 0113 244 1400

sanofi-aventis
www.sanofi-aventis.co.uk
Tel: 01483 505 515

Servier Laboratories
www.servier.co.uk
Tel: 01753 666 409

Takeda UK
www.takeda.co.uk
Tel: 01628 537 900

Wockhardt UK
www.wockhardt.co.uk
Tel: 01978 661 261

Medical

MedicAlert®
www.medicalert.org.uk
Tel: 0800 581 420

Coeliac disease
www.coeliac.org.uk
Tel: 0870 444 8804

National Institute of Clinical Excellence (NICE)
www.nice.org.uk
Tel: 0845 003 7780 (London)
Tel: 0845 003 7780 (Manchester)
For national gold standard guidelines and recommendations.

Insulin pumps

INPUT
www.input.me.uk
A patient-led support group for people using insulin pumps.

School

Directgov
www.directgov.co.uk
Official government website; link for application for special educational needs and disability living allowance.

Bullying

www.bullying.co.uk
For young people and their parents coping with bullying.

Sports and recreation

Cinema Exhibitors' Association Ltd (CEA)
www.ceacard.co.uk
Tel: 0845 123 1292

UK Sport Diving Medical Committee
www.uksdmc.co.uk

Runsweet
www.runsweet.com

Weight issues

Eating Disorders Association
www.edauk.com
Tel: 0845 634 7650
Advice for people aged 18 and under.

Weight Concern
www.weightconcern.com
Tel: 020 7679 1853

Employment

Civil Aviation Authority
www.caa.co.uk
Tel: 01293 573725

www.hse.gov.uk/workplacehealth
Tel: 0845 345 0055
For advice on Health and Safety at work

Careers office
www.careersadvice.direct.gov.uk

Careers in defence
www.mod.uk/DefenceInternet

Driving

Driver and Vehicle Licensing Agency (DVLA)
www.dvla.gov.uk
www.dft.gov.uk/drivingforwork
www.dft.gov.uk/pgr/regional/taxis/taxiandprivatehirevehiclelic
Tel: 020 7944 8300

Index

Have you found **Diabetes Through the Looking Glass** useful and practical? If so, you may be interested in other books from **Class Publishing**.

Type 1 Diabetes: Answers at your fingertips £14.99

Dr Charles Fox and Dr Anne Kilvert

This practical handbook makes it easy for you to learn more about your diabetes – and the more you know the easier it will be to manage. Written by medical experts, the book offers practical advice on every aspect of living with diabetes, presented in a user-friendly question and answer format. It guides you through all the medical terminology you are likely to encounter, and shows you exactly what to do if an emergency occurs.

'I have no hesitation in commending this book.'
– Sir Steve Redgrave, Vice President, Diabetes UK

Type 1 Diabetes in children, adolescents and young adults £19.99

Dr Ragnar Hanas

Dr Ragnar Hanas shows you step-by-step how to become an expert in your own diabetes. It has been written not only for the person with diabetes and their parents but also for members of the diabetes care team.

'It is an incredible book, which deals in depth with every detail of diabetes care in young people and it never ducks any issues.'
– Dr Charles Fox, Consultant Physician at Northampton General Hospital

Effective Management of Bladder and Bowel problems in Children £29.99

Liz Bonner and Mandy Wells (Editors)

This comprehensive text explores all continence problems in children and gives practical, easy-to-adopt guidance on how they can be controlled and managed in the clinical and community setting. Chapters are written by leading practitioners from a range of disciplines: nursing, medicine, surgery, psychology and education.

Eczema: Answers at your fingertips £14.99

Dr Tim Mitchell and Alison Hepplewhite

With answers to hundreds of questions on every aspect of living with eczema, this book will help you find ways to manage your own eczema – or that of your child.

'What a joy to have a new book which is medically accurate, wide ranging and practical in its approach.'
– Margaret Cox, Chief Executive, National Eczema Society

Asthma: Answers at your fingertips £17.99

Dr Mark Levy, Trisha Weller and Professor Sean Hilton

Contains over 250 real questions from people with asthma and their families – answered by three medical experts. This handbook contains up-to-date, medically accurate and practical advice on living with asthma.

'A helpful and clearly written book.'
– Dr Martyn Partridge, Chief Medical Adviser, National Asthma Campaign

Allergies: Answers at your fingertips £17.99

Dr Joanne Clough

A fully updated edition that gives you clear and concise information on allergies including what they are, how they develop and (most important of all) how to deal with them. This authoritative handbook covers a broad range of allergic problems including asthma, eczema, dermatitis, hay fever, food allergies, coeliac disease and anaphylaxis.

'Excellent first-hand guidance.'
– Professor Stephen Holgate, Southampton General Hospital

PRIORITY ORDER FORM

Cut out or photocopy this form and send it (post free in the UK) to:

Class Publishing Priority Service, FREEPOST 16705,
Macmillan Distribution, Basingstoke, RG21 6ZZ
Tel: 01256 302 699   Fax: 01256 812 558

Please send me urgently (tick below)
Post included price per copy (UK only)

☐ **Diabetes Through the Looking Glass** (ISBN 978 1 85959 209 0) **£20.99**

☐ **Type 1 Diabetes in children, adolescents and young adults**
(ISBN 978 1 85959 173 4) **£22.99**

☐ **Type 1 Diabetes: Answers at your fingertips**
(ISBN 978 1 85959 175 8) **£17.99**

☐ **Effective Management of Bladder and Bowel Problems in**
Children (ISBN 978 1 85959 165 9) **£32.99**

☐ **Eczema: Answers at your fingertips** (ISBN 978 1 85959 125 3) **£17.99**

☐ **Asthma: Answers at your fingertips** (ISBN 978 1 85959 111 6) **£20.99**

☐ **Allergies: Answers at your fingertips** (ISBN 978 1 85959 147 5) **£20.99**

TOTAL:

Easy ways to pay:

Cheque: I enclose a cheque payable to Class Publishing for: _____

Credit card: please debit my ☐ Mastercard ☐ Visa ☐ Amex

Number: _____ Expiry date: _____

Name: _____

My address for delivery is: _____

_____

Town _____

County_____ Postcode _____

Telephone number (in case of query) _____

Credit card billing address if different from above _____

_____

Town _____

County_____ Postcode _____

Class Publishing's guarantee: remember that if, for any reason, you are not satisfied with these books, we will refund all your money, without any questions asked. Prices and VAT rates may be altered for reasons beyond our control.

The following four pages are taken from our sixth edition of *Type 1 Diabetes: Answers at your fingertips*

1 | What is diabetes?

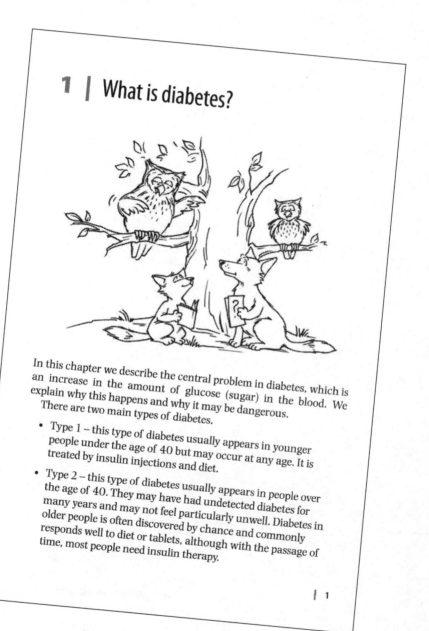

In this chapter we describe the central problem in diabetes, which is an increase in the amount of glucose (sugar) in the blood. We explain why this happens and why it may be dangerous. There are two main types of diabetes.

- Type 1 – this type of diabetes usually appears in younger people under the age of 40 but may occur at any age. It is treated by insulin injections and diet.

- Type 2 – this type of diabetes usually appears in people over the age of 40. They may have had undetected diabetes for many years and may not feel particularly unwell. Diabetes in older people is often discovered by chance and commonly responds well to diet or tablets, although with the passage of time, most people need insulin therapy.

There are other rare types of diabetes, which we also mention in this chapter.

WHAT HAPPENS IN DIABETES?

The pancreas is a gland situated in the upper part of the abdomen and connected by a fine tube to the intestine (see Figure 1.1). One of its functions is to release into the gut digestive juices, which are mixed with food soon after it leaves the stomach.

These digestive juices are needed to break down food and help it be absorbed into the body. This part of the pancreas has nothing to do with diabetes.

The pancreas also produces a number of hormones which are released directly into the bloodstream, unlike the digestive juices which pass into the intestine. The most important of these hormones is insulin, a shortage of which causes diabetes. The other important

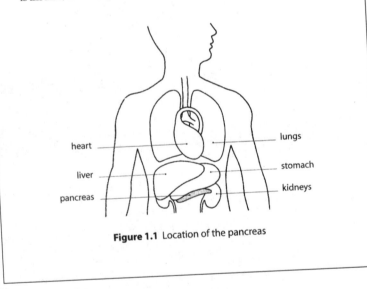

Figure 1.1 Location of the pancreas

[Pages shown smaller than actual size]

292

hormone produced by the pancreas is glucagon, which has the opposite action to insulin and may be used in correcting serious hypos. 'Hypo' is short for hypoglycaemia, meaning low blood glucose. See the section *Hypos* in Chapter 3. Both hormones come from a part of the pancreas called the islets of Langerhans, which are scattered throughout the pancreas.

Why does the body need insulin?

Without insulin the body cannot make use of the food we eat. Food is broken down in the stomach and intestine into simple chemicals, such as glucose and fatty acids, which provide fuel for all the activities of the body. These simple chemicals also provide building blocks for growth or replacing worn out parts, and any extra is stored for later use. In diabetes, food is broken down as normal but, because of the shortage of insulin (or sometimes because insulin does not work properly), excess glucose cannot be stored and builds up in the bloodstream. When glucose rises above a certain level, it spills into the urine through the kidneys.

The liver plays a dual role in processing food. It converts simple chemicals into complex substances which are then stored for future use and it also allows breakdown of these stores when they are needed for fuel. This process is controlled by insulin. For example, in the absence of insulin, glycogen (starch) is broken down into glucose, which pours out of the liver into the bloodstream (and then into the urine). Insulin switches off this outpouring of glucose and causes the glucose to be stored as glycogen. Thus insulin ensures that a perfect balance is kept between the production of glucose and its storage, and in this way it maintains the blood glucose at a normal level. Insulin plays other important roles, such as allowing glucose to get into other parts of the body to be used as a fuel, and regulating the processing of amino acids and fatty acids, which are the breakdown products of protein and fat.

For ordering details for the sixth edition of *Type 1 Diabetes: Answers at your fingertips*, please see our order form ...

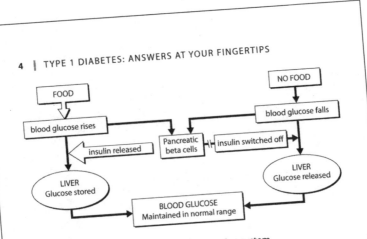

Figure 1.2 Insulin production system

What happens to insulin production in diabetes?

In people who do not have diabetes, insulin is produced in the pancreas and released into the blood as soon as the blood glucose level starts to rise after eating. Insulin travels straight from the pancreas to the liver where it has the important role of regulating glucose production and the storage of glucose as glycogen. The level of glucose in the blood then falls and, as it does so, insulin production is switched off, allowing glucose to be released from stores in the liver (see Figure 1.2). In people who do not have diabetes this sensitive system keeps the amount of glucose in the blood at a steady level.

In diabetes this process is faulty. People with Type 2 diabetes can still produce some insulin but not in adequate amounts to keep the blood glucose level normal. This is because their insulin does not work properly (a condition called 'insulin resistance'). People with Type 1 diabetes have little or no insulin of their own and need injections of insulin to try to keep the blood glucose level normal. Even if given four or five times a day, injected insulin is not as efficient at regulating blood glucose as the pancreas, which responds instantly to small changes in blood glucose by switching the insulin supply on or off.

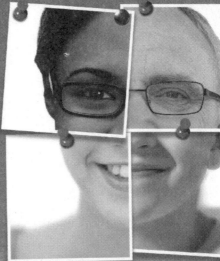
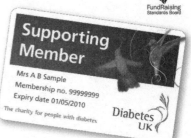

Become a Friend of the Juvenile Diabetes Research Foundation

Juvenile Diabetes Research Foundation (JDRF) exists to find the cure for Type 1 diabetes and its complications. It is the world's leading charitable funder of Type 1 diabetes research.

JDRF was founded in the USA 40 years ago, by a small group of parents of children with Type 1 diabetes. They knew that insulin was not the cure for the condition and recognised that the only way to find the cure was through research.

As a result, over the last 40 years, JDRF volunteers and staff around the world have been responsible for raising more than £650 million to support Type 1 diabetes research. Projects that are funded by JDRF aim to prevent, treat and cure the condition and its serious and debilitating complications.

Thanks to research, JDRF has contributed to some of the key advances in the field. This new understanding has made a lasting difference to the lives of people with Type 1 diabetes. For example, in 1990 the idea of transplanting islets routinely was unthinkable. JDRF funded research allowed scientists in Canada to develop an effective way of transplanting islets from the pancreas of an organ donor to a person with Type 1 diabetes. Once implanted, the islets make and release insulin in response to glucose levels. Researchers have shown that islet transplantation can positively impact the lives of people who are unable to manage their Type 1 diabetes through conventional treatments.

JDRF also funded the first independent clinical trial examining whether continuous glucose monitors could help people with Type 1 diabetes to achieve better blood sugar control. This ground-breaking trial proved the effectiveness of these devices, and the results of this trial are already helping more people to access this technology, improving quality of life and reducing the risk of complications.

In the UK, JDRF is proud to have some of the most promising research, right on its doorstep. The Artificial Pancreas Project at the University of Cambridge is one of these cutting edge studies. The research aims to develop a system that can automatically regulate blood glucose levels. This system focuses on 'closing the loop' between two existing technologies – insulin pumps and continuous glucose monitors. Getting these devices to 'talk' to each other would minimise or even remove the need for human intervention in the day-to-day management of Type 1 diabetes.

Another important project in the UK is the JDRF Collaborative Centre for Diabetes – Genes, Autoimmunity and Prevention. This project seeks to unravel the links between Type 1 diabetes risk genes and the changes in the immune system that lead to the development of Type 1 diabetes. The knowledge gained through this research could potentially help us to develop treatments that prevent high risk individuals from ever developing Type 1 diabetes in the first place.

Only research will find the cure. JDRF exists to fund that research.

Every day hundreds of scientists around the world are working towards a shared goal: to find the cure for Type 1 diabetes. But it's not just scientists who will make this dream a reality. Even 40 years after the charity's inception, JDRF's work is still driven by those affected by Type 1 diabetes. Most of JDRF's staff and volunteers have a connection to the condition and it is this that gives us the dedication to find the cure.

We believe that finding the cure for Type 1 diabetes is only a matter of time and money. This is where you can help.

The more money we raise, the more research we can fund and the faster we can find the cure. You can help by becoming a Friend of JDRF. You will be joining a network of the charity's most loyal supporters. When you sign up as a Friend of JDRF, we promise to keep you updated with the research developments you are helping to fund.

You will receive JDRF's quarterly magazine Diabetes Breakthrough and JDRF International's magazine Countdown. You will also receive invitations to JDRF Research Open Days and other events, as well as a special quarterly Friends' e-bulletin.

£60, or just £5 a month, could help fund an hour of research.

Signing up is easy. All you need to do is make a regular donation to JDRF, and we will do the rest. Please contact us on 020 7713 2030 and help make research a reality today.

Join us in finding the cure.

Juvenile Diabetes Research Foundation
19 Angel Gate
City Road
London EC1V 2PT
(020) 7713 2030
info@jdrf.org.uk
www.jdrf.org.uk

Registered as a charity in England and Wales (No.295716) and in Scotland (No.SC040123)